The Number One Book of
Pregnancy and Fitness Questions

By
Alexandra Allred

For
Kerri, Katie and Tommy

THANK YOU!

The Number One Book of Pregnancy and Fitness Questions © 2013 Alexandra Allred

ISBN-13   978-1491216576
ISBN-10   1491216573

Published with Allredbooks
Distributed through CreateSpace, on-demand publishing, LLC

The Number One Book Of Pregnancy & Fitness Questions

By
Alexandra Allred

Table of Contents

Chapter 5 - What's My Problem
1. The Hormones Effect: Mood Swings, Morning Sickness, Constipation, and Heartburn
2. Anemia: Fatigue and Dizziness
3. High Blood Pressure
4. Thyroid
5. Hypoglycemia
6. Fertility and Miscarriages
7. Vitamins – Or Lack Thereof
8. Your Team

Chapter 6 -- Already An Athlete?
1. What Will the Neighbors Say?
2. Acclimated Muscles
3. Check with your Team, Update the Doctors
4. Advice for the Super Fit
5. It's Not a Contest
6. I'm in Shape! Why Am I So Tired?!

Chapter 7 – The Couch Potato
1. The Pregnancy.org Dream Team
2. "I'm Fat" and "I'm Lazy": Today's Motto
3. Let's Get Real about Working Out
4. True Confessions of a Recovering Potato
5. Building Muscle

Chapter 8 – Why Even Bother
1. The benefits of exercise for labor and delivery
2. The beneficial baby
3. Baby Blues
4. Muscle Memory
5. Better Moms, Better Babies
6. Team Baby

Part II: Working Out or Finding Your Sport While Pregnant

Chapter 9: The Controlled Workout
1. The Machines: StairMaster, Elliptical, Treadmill, and Cycling
2. The Traditional 50-minute Cardio Class: Kickboxing, Aerobics, Step, Bootcamp, and Modern Dance
3. The Pros and Cons of Yoga
4. The Joys of Walking and Swimming

Be Advised!

Before beginning any exercise routine you must consult your primary physician and OB/GYN.

The questions and answers offered here are sample questions taken from the fitness website www.pregnancy.org. The publisher, author and pregnancy organization are in no way liable for injury. Only you and your physician(s) know your physical conditioning and medical history. While we encourage fitness, you must always be careful and cautious in your exercise routines. Please discuss any and all training and nutritional changes with a medical expert. Keep your doctor apprised of your routine as you progress.

Introduction

From the start, let me say this: no one is perfect. Yet, we drive ourselves nuts looking at pictures of touched-up, airbrushed supermodels and compare ourselves to the impossible. Even though supermodels have confessed, "I don't even look like this!" we still compare and scrutinize. Why do we do this?

Nothing but nothing is more annoying than a skinny celebrity who has never known a fat day in her life making a fitness video. Who wants to take advice from a woman who has built a career on having an almost perfect body with airbrushed photos of her in undies and bikinis?

It is important for you to know then that I built my own career on the fact that I never knew fudge I could walk away from, I live to eat rather than eat to live, and my athletic career was simply a reasonable reaction to justify my voracious appetite. I love to eat. Fortunately for me, I love to workout and sweat so this supported my bread-loving habits. And while pregnant – though I in no way endorse this behavior – I once ate an entire jar of Smuckers raspberry jam, complete with Hershey's chocolate syrup on top. It was so sweet, it actually took the skin off the roof of my mouth, but I kept eating. It was painfully delicious. Needless to say, I paid the price for my sweet tooth.

While many women quietly attempt to regain their pre-pregnancy state after having a baby, trying all the latest diets or work out fads, I had exactly one month to get into some kind of shape before returning to the Olympic Training Center for the U.S. women's bobsled team and just seven months before I would be wearing a spandex bodysuit on live television at the World Cup in Calgary. Hey, no pressure!

I am well aware of poor body image, weight gain, mother's apron, and post partum depression. For those reasons (and more), this may be the easiest book I've ever written. I've lived it. I lived the questions and concerns, the fear of working out, and the benefits of a great exercise program all described in these pages. My first pregnancy was one of worry. I worried about my weight gain, my diet, and working out. Each time I huffed and puffed, I stopped working out for fear of harming my baby. As a result of not knowing how much was too much, I just quit working out completely.

During my second pregnancy, I was working with a research team while I trained for the U.S. women's bobsled team. Between runs for the bathroom, morning sickness, and fatigue, I was running 30-, 60-, and 100-meter sprint intervals, squatting 200-300 lbs., performing plyometrics, running the stairs in football stadiums, and jogging longer distances for stamina. I was pushing 400 lbs. bobsleds on dry-land tracks, throwing shot put, and lifting weights.

The renowned obstetric researcher and professor of reproductive biology, Dr. James Clapp, III, had never studied my kind of physical routine before. Clapp had been studying the correlation between athletics and healthy pregnancies, examining the intensity of many types of exercise from aerobic dancers to marathon runners. But he'd never studied anyone who was lifting the amount of weights I was lifting or performing the plyometrics I was doing. When his team invited me to train at their MetroHealth Hospital in Cleveland, Ohio, I leapt at the opportunity.

I believed I could make the women's bobsled team but I was also pregnant for the second time and was suddenly uncertain as to how much I could actually do. Throughout my first pregnancy and into my second, all I had read in various magazines and books was to not allow my heart rate to exceed 140 beats per minute.

The 140 bpm guideline did not take into account how conditioned an athlete may already be prior to pregnancy. There was never any mention of inner core temperature. Elite athletes found these limiting guidelines frustrating and many Olympic athletes have reported simply giving up, overeating and gaining more weight than they wish they had during their pregnancies.

For me, Clapp's research was a dream come true. While under his supervision, I was hooked up to heart and fetal monitors, EKG leads, a rectal thermometer, and oxygen mask. And away we went!!

While I learned about my heart rate, recovery rate, the baby's activity during exercise and after, Dr. Clapp studied my placenta – more specifically, the growth of placenta as a result of exercise.

The placenta is a membranous organ that lines the uterine wall and helps protect and cradle the baby. It exists for the sole purpose of getting nutrients and oxygen from the mother's body into the baby's body. Clapp believed that the largest placentas have been produced due to vigorous workout programs during the critical period of placenta growth. Further, he believed that exercise produces larger placentas, which offer healthier, stronger wombs and, thus, healthier pregnancies and babies.

On September 25, 1994, the first ever U.S. women's bobsled team was named. The world was stunned to learn that the woman who took gold for the U.S. Nationals was four and a half months pregnant. Who are we kidding? I was stunned! I was named *Athlete of the Year* by the United States Olympic Committee and began answering phone calls and letters from around the world about how I did what I did. But the other surprise was that the woman who took silver, Liz Parr-Smestad, was also pregnant! At three and four months pregnant, Liz and I made sports history.

After retiring from bobsledding in 1998, I went on to earn my second black belt in martial arts. I was also pregnant for a third time and teaching kickboxing. This pregnancy centered more on stretches, martial arts moves and cardio kickbox routines. I met and worked with some of the greatest martial artists today such as Billy Blanks, the creator of Tae Bo; Ernie Reyes and Jhoon Rhee, the fathers of modern day tae kwon do.

Over the years, I've done a number of interviews in both print media and on television with the same results. Women committed to exercise wanted to know how I knew what I could do and how much was too much. PBS did a feature on our training regimen while Clapp's research team entered into the second phase of the research project: testing my bobsled baby when she turned five years old in support of the theory that babies of exercising moms have better verbal and cognitive skills, lower body fat, and higher/better coordination. All true. Lean, muscular, athletic, outgoing, and highly intelligent, Katie Allred is the poster child for why mothers-to-be should work out.

But it was not until I connected with www.pregnancy.org and began to answer questions over from, quite literally, around the world that I realized how greatly this book was needed. Answering questions about various fitness and dietary questions from around the United States, the United Kingdom, India, Latin America, and the Slavic nations, the pregnancy.org team has busily tried to dispel myths from "Should I drink coconut milk" to "should I stand on my head after sex" to conceive. We've offered advice on better nutritional habits, as well as answers to fitness questions about skiing, hiking, yoga, soccer, jogging, horseback riding, aerobics, weight lifting, and more. We've tackled issues on breastfeeding, morning sickness, coffee drinking habits, stretch marks, and c-sections. And we've repeatedly informed the pregnancy public about inner core temperature – something that physicians still seem to be relatively uninformed about.

Personally, I have lectured on the subject of inner core temperature to more trainers, more physicians, more certified instructors, and more coaches than I could possibly count. But I have also counseled women on the idea that pregnancy is not a life sentence to an out-of-shape or overweight body. You can get into shape while pregnant. Yes, you can! And, as you will read, most gold-medal Olympic athletes (who are also mothers) will tell you that they returned to athletics stronger, faster, and more determined after having a baby. After. Motherhood, they contend, makes you better.

Whether you are pregnant or planning to be, this book is designed to educate you as to how to work out safely and happily. As you read questions and answers from around the world, from women who are underweight or clinically obese, of Olympic stature or completely sedentary, pregnant for the first time or into a sixth pregnancy, you will find a common thread. They all want to be stronger, healthier, and happier for their baby and for themselves.

That's the goal here. Pregnancy is not an end to healthy living but, rather, the beginning to a new and better world. As the saying goes, "When momma's not happy, ain't nobody happy." I'll add to that. When momma's strong and kicking booty, the possibilities for both momma and baby are endless!

Chapter One
Getting Started: Let's Get Real

"Hi. I just found out I'm pregnant and I would like a good exercise program to keep in shape but not so intense to hurt the baby. Could you help me please?

Sound familiar? Or …

"I am overweight and I started a fitness program a few weeks before I found out I was pregnant. I have heard people say you can continue a fitness routine that your body was used to. But my body wasn't use to any exercise. Can I continue working out or do I need to take it easy? I am really concerned about gaining weight, and want to get my body in better shape."

Or ….

"Hello, I just found out I'm pregnant (not my first) and am not sure about a fitness routine. After my last pregnancy, I worked out six days a week very strenuously for about a year, but have fallen out of my routine the past few months. How much can I do now that I'm pregnant? I've also gained some weight back, and really want to keep my weight gain during pregnancy under check."

Or, the very popular question of …

"I just found out I'm pregnant but I'm scared because I know I'm overweight. Can I be on a diet while I'm pregnant?"

1. The Number One Question

Hands down, the most commonly asked question I get from around the world is about weight. "I just found out I'm pregnant. How can I get into shape before my body starts to change?" Or, phrased differently, "I just found out I'm pregnant but I'm overweight. Can I lose weight while I'm pregnant?"

Nothing will send women scrambling for a fitness program faster than an upcoming wedding, bathing suit season, and pregnancy. Yes, you can get into shape while pregnant but there are several "but" factors that must be addressed. To properly answer those questions, we have to establish a few safety rules. Whether you are a seasoned athlete, the dedicated weekend warrior on a mountain bike, or have never intentionally burned a calorie but now want to workout, you have to take some precautionary steps. Here we go:

Question:
"I am overweight and I started a fitness routine a few weeks before I found out I was pregnant. I have heard people say you can continue a fitness routine that

your body was used to. My body wasn't used to any exercise. Can I continue working out or do I need to take it easy? I am really concerned about gaining more weight, and want to get my body into better shape.

Answer:

Yes, it is true that your body becomes acclimated to a workout routine and can easily handle it during pregnancy if this is an activity your body is already used to. Experts worry about women who are newly pregnant and jump into a new exercise routine because of the sudden strain it may present to her body. Unfortunately, others have taken this guideline to mean it is better to do nothing if you've been sedentary.

Let's break down your situation. You've committed yourself to working out (good for you!) but because you have not been able to adjust to a new routine, you must first speak to your personal physician and your OB/GYN. Because I do not know what your medical history is, it is important that you have medical permission to exercise. You need to let your doctor know what your plans are in terms of exercise.

Too many women focus on the weight issue rather than the health issue. Because the reality is this: unless you are clinically obese, you will gain weight during a healthy pregnancy. (*see Chapter Two on obesity and weight gain for more information).

After getting the green light for exercise, you need to meet with a trainer and nutritionist. Even if money is too tight for regular visits, most gyms offer a $30-ish fee for a one-time meeting. You need to talk to someone about the kinds of exercise you have been or plan on doing. It is important that a professional help you with proper body posture and positioning so that you do not hurt yourself while lifting weights or performing specific physical activities. This may sound silly but we see people every day who are doing more harm than good on their non-pregnant frames by poor posture or movement. I cringe to think of pregnant women doing this.

Again, if money is an issue, meet with a trainer just once a month to check on your progress and body position. As your body changes so, too, will your movements. Quite unconsciously, you will readjust your stances because of your growing belly. We want to protect your back, core, and muscle groups from injury.

By seeing a nutritionist, you can take a hard look at what you eat and drink. A nutritionist can figure what you are and aren't doing in preparation of your baby in terms of proper diet. Again, far too many women use pregnancy as a license to eat, eat, eat while others panic about weight gain and consume too few calories.

Studies have shown that how you exercise and what you eat really impact the next ten months and how you feel. As corny as it sounds, knowledge is power. You will feel more confident about working out when you are informed.

Question:

I just found out I am pregnant and I would like a good exercise program to keep in shape but not so intense to hurt the baby. Could you please help?

Answer:

You are wise to want to get in/stay in shape. But before I can advise you to work out you must first speak with your personal physician and OB/GYN about your current health, physical activity level, and pregnancy. Because I don't know your medical history, it's important that you speak to your physicians first. The easy answer here is to say walking and/or swimming are good, low-impact exercise programs to start with. But you may be beyond that level. The best thing for you to do is meet with a trainer who can properly assess your physical abilities and conditioning. Even if you cannot afford a gym membership, this trainer should be able to give you a safe workout routine according to your abilities where you can exercise at home. But this is where I require some work from you. Do not randomly pick a trainer and hope for the best.

Be sure the trainer you choose is qualified to work with a pregnant client. Do not be afraid to ask for credentials and call on them. Share this information with your OB/GYN. A great question to ask your trainer to determine if she or he knows anything about working out a pregnant client is the almighty inner core temperature question. Ask, "Do you know what that is? How hot can a pregnant woman get while working out?" The answer: Your baby is one degree Celsius hotter than you are but has no way to sweat. Therefore, it is suggested that your own body temperature not exceed 101 degrees F. If your potential trainer does not know the answer, find someone else.

Do not be surprised if your trainer instantly offers you information about 140 beats per minute rather than the inner core temperature. Again, most certified trainers know very little about the inner core temperature. You may wind up teaching a few things to your own trainer!

A solid trainer should be able to give you a workout program in the gym or at home. By working with a trainer, even just once a month, this insures a safer workout with more effective movements and the peace of mind you need to have fun while you get in shape and prepare for the physical event of your life!

Question:

Hello, I just found out I'm pregnant (not my first) and am not sure about a fitness program. After my last pregnancy, I worked out six days a week very strenuously for about a year, but have fallen out of my routine the past few months. How much can I do now that I'm pregnant? I've also gained some weight back and really want to keep my weight gain during pregnancy under check.

Answer:

Muscle memory is a great thing and no doubt, you will be surprised how quickly your body will respond to working out again. However, you must check first with your doctor before working out. Many women assume that because a first pregnancy was healthy and they could workout, that they are safe to do the same during the second and third. Most likely, your physician will give you a big thumbs up for exercise but let's be safe and ask first. After you've discussed your previous pregnancies and current health with him or her, then talk about the exercise program you are most interested in.

If you had, for example, been going to the gym five times a week, attending three cardio classes and lifting weights (light) on alternate days, you would be safe to continue this workout regime. Because your body would be acclimated to the muscle strain/stress of lifting weights (again, light weights) and the cardio, you could simply continue with a few tweaks along the way. Again, this is contingent on doctor permission.

If you have never worked out, I would start you with walking (holding 1 or 2 lbs. hand weights) and lift weights with a trainer. It would be imperative that you begin training with someone who can monitor your responses to weights and cardio routines as you start out. Because there is no history, I would need to know how your body reacted to said workouts. Even if you are limited in funds, it is always worth it to pay for one to three workouts with a professional. So, we come to your question. You have worked out and know that you can handle a pretty strenuous routine. This is a great beginning. If you 1) are given permission to workout and 2) start slowly (recommended that you have at least two training sessions with a professional just to get your started), you should have no problems returning to light runs, walking, treadmill, StairMaster and/or aerobic classes with circuit training.

*RED FLAG!

I am, however, always concerned to hear women talk about weight issues when they become pregnant. It is expected that you will gain weight and you need to celebrate this point in your life. This doesn't mean you should eat non-stop and gain 100 pounds, but know that genetics play a huge part in each pregnancy. Do NOT look around at other pregnant women and compare yourself. Do NOT compare yourself to the pregnant models (who may or may not even be pregnant) or listen to other people talk about the ideal weight. This is an issue between you and your doctor.

Using myself as an example, I gained 60 lbs with my first pregnancy and didn't really workout. I was scared about what I could do and decided nothing was better than something.

Baby #2 was a different story as I was training for the US women's bobsled team and, working with a research group. I was working with a team of professional trainers six days a week, four to five hours a day! I was squatting over 300 lbs., running sprint intervals at national level times, running stadium steps and pushing a

400 lbs. sled. I won the national title and had a very healthy baby girl. My labor was fast, easy. My recovery was so fast I was back in the gym in record time and guess what? I gained a total of 65 pounds.

Because of muscle memory and my dedication to working out, the weight came off SLOWLY while I was nursing. But the most important thing was my health and that of my little girl.

With baby #3, I was training for my black belt and teaching kickbox classes. I performed countless kicks, deep leg lunges, squats, and punches. It was a happy medium between my first and second pregnancy. And guess what? I gained about 50 pounds.

While pregnant, your overall health and that of your baby's is all that matters. Once the baby is born, you can focus more fully on your weight but while pregnant, think of this as your Olympic event – to make the best and healthiest baby ever.

But be smart. Talk to your doctor, interview a few personal trainers who have worked with pregnant clients, find a workout buddy, and exercise for health.

Don't look at the scale!!!

2. Get the Green Light from Your Doctor

No farmer's wife, who is a mother, ought to be allowed to do the washing of the family [laundry]; it is perilous to any woman who has not a vigorous constitution.
- The Guide Board to Health, Peace
and Competence, 1869

We've come a long way, baby. But before you begin any exercise program, you must speak to your doctor about your "constitution."

Question:
I feel great! I don't need to talk to my doctor. I've been working out all along! Why would I need to talk to my doctor if everything is already fine?

Answer:
There are two things you can always count on while pregnant – constant doctor appointments and constant trips to the bathroom. Both feel like endless exercises in futility but both are greatly needed.

My theory is this: Each time you wake at 12 a.m., 2 a.m., and 4 a.m. to the frustrating realization that you need to go to the bathroom, this is Mother Nature's way of preparing you for the fact that once baby is born, you will be waking up just as many times throughout the night to tend to and feed your newborn.

Going to the doctor, keeping updated and accurate file of information with him or her is preparing you for all the trips you will be taking once you have your newborn. Believe me, you will be making many necessary trips to the pediatrician once your baby is born. So, keeping in check with your OB/GYN and telling him or her (and the staff) what you are doing is all part of the process. It keeps you safe and in practice for what is to come.

But beyond that, there may be medical conditions that you should be made aware of such as high blood pressure, diabetes, or even a torn or strained abdominal muscle from a previous c-section. You never know. It is always better for both you and baby to be safe and prepared.

Throughout this book, there is mention of the training team I had while pregnant and training for a national team. My team was invaluable to me, offering great peace of mind. Included in that team were my physicians. While I trusted my trainers and worked hard, I also included my doctors on how I ate, slept, and trained. They were very much a part of my long-term goals.

You should also make a list of your long-term goals to present to your doctor. Think about what it is you realistically want and need. Realistically being the key word. If you are 5'1", it is unlikely that you will carry your baby in the way that 6'3" professional volleyball player and model Gabrielle Reece has. But if you want to get into better shape, develop muscle, and build your cardiovascular threshold, this is a realistic goal. Whether you are planning to get pregnant, are already pregnant, or wondering about your fitness routine post-baby, make a list.

Hoping to Get Pregnant
   1. Discuss current health status with doctor.
   2. Address any potential medical problems or limitations that a trainer needs to know about.
   3. Are you overweight or underweight? Is this an issue that may need to be addressed as you try to conceive?
   4. Discuss your current fitness level. Share your fitness goals with your doctor. For example, do you simply wish to lose weight or are you hoping to run 3 miles or build upper body strength?

Pregnant with New Goals
   1. Discuss your current health status with both your personal physician and OB/GYN.
   2. Address any potential medical problems or limitations that a trainer needs to know about before working out.
   3. Have an honest conversation about your weight. If you are over or underweight, these are issues that need to be addressed with both your doctors and a nutritionist to evaluate your present dietary habits.
   4. Share your personal fitness goals with your doctor. Be honest. Be realistic. This is not the time to worry about weight. Focus on better health and better stamina throughout the pregnancy. But this doesn't mean you cannot set fitness goals as well!

3. Home at the Gym and Training at Home

"Lose weight now!" "Get a flat tummy in three days!"

Now that I have your attention …don't you just hate those headlines? But in this fast food world we occupy, where everything is instant, why not lose weight instantly and effortlessly? You can get instant credit, instant grits and instant service, so why not instant weight loss?

This month, like every month, every men's and women's health magazine promises new wonder diets, new sure-fire training techniques, and the new miracle pills that claim to burn fat while you sleep. Everyone wants to have the perfect body, but with limited effort. While headlines scream radical weight loss programs, your belly is beginning to swell. Despite your best efforts, worry sets in. What if I never get in shape again?

A recent poll conducted by Ladies Home Journal revealed that more than 50 percent of the women polled would give up a year of life if they could attain their ideal weight and stay there. A year?!

They'd give up a year of life, but won't give up 30 minutes a day just to work out?

Whether you are working out in the gym or training at home, you can safely begin a training program that will fit your lifestyle. But you have to be committed and honest with yourself.

The cold reality is this: only 20 percent of Americans work out more than 100 days a year. Getting started in a fitness routine is the hardest aspect of training.

The Gym

Whether you are already a member of a gym or a first-timer, introduce yourself to the head trainer at the gym and explain that you are pregnant and want to work (if only one time) with a trainer who is well versed in training pregnant clients. Throughout the book, you will find a wide variety of tips about training with various equipment, but here are some additional things to think about while training at the gym:

Question:

"I've read that saunas, hot tubs, and hot baths may be related to early miscarriage. I'm in my 5th week and have stopped attending my water aerobics class because the pool they use is a heated pool at around 88 degrees F. I've been exercising consistently before becoming pregnant, so this does fall under the category of "something I did before pregnancy" but the water temperature concerns me. Is it okay?"

Answer:

Working out in a pool of 88 degree F is a "comfort" temp for people working out and poses no danger to your baby. Higher temperatures, however, worry experts as there may be a correlation between miscarriages and high temperatures. Hot tubs, typically ranging in the area of 101 to 104 degree F, pose a danger as it may raise your own inner core temperature of the typical 98.6 F to a dangerous level. But there is the additional concern that hot tubs can be a breeding ground for all kinds of bacteria.

It is not recommended that you use heated baths while pregnant. However, the heated pool of 88 degrees can offer a safe workout that is easy on your joints. Water aerobics can be one of the very best workouts you can do while pregnant.

Question:

I'm ready to start a gym membership now that I'm pregnant. What should I do when I get there? Do you have any suggestions?

Answer:

You bet. Begin slowly. Because I do not know your medical background and suspect you may not be a regular exerciser, you need to speak with a trainer. I want to ensure the safest route of training and urge that you begin by working one-on-one with a trainer who will make sure you learn proper form and technique when you lift and perform cardiovascular exercises. How you move, stand, lift, position your legs and upper torso mean the difference in how much you can lift, how quickly your muscles will respond to a fitness program and your own personal safety.

I want to be sure that you are not so sore that you are too afraid (or hurt) to return to the gym. Be sure to talk to communicate with your trainer – tell him or her when something is too difficult or too heavy. Don't try to be "tough."

In addition to working with a trainer, there are three additional safety measures you can take to ensure better success. Drink lots of water, listen to your body, and use a rectal thermometer.

1. Water: It sounds so simple and we are all conditioned to hearing/reading about the importance of water but the majority of Americans are clinically dehydrated. We are drinking everything we can get our hands (and lips) on except water. Water also helps prevent morning sickness – something you may be experiencing early in pregnancy – which often makes women drink even less water and become more sedentary as working out doesn't sound nearly so appealing as curling up on the couch. Water will energize you, help your workouts, and prevent morning sickness.
2. Listen to your body: As your belly swells and your baby grows, other body parts will be changing as well. Your joints will loosen, feet and breasts may

swell. You know the difference between feeling lazy or tired and something hurting. There are no multi-million dollar sport contracts on the line and no Hollywood movie demanding that you work out like a fiend. If something doesn't feel right, back off. Listen to and respect what your body is going through. Sometimes, the best medicine is a nap. The weights can wait!

3. Rectal thermometer. Icky-ooh-ey. I know. I know. But it is the best way to make sure you do not overheat while working out. Your baby's temperature is one degree Celsius higher than your own but your baby has no sweating mechanism. If you overheat, so does your baby without the benefit of sweating – a natural cooling response. Making sure your inner core temperature does not exceed 101 degree F., you should dash off to the bathroom and take your inner core temperature. As you will read more about this safety training method, you will understand how it offers peace of mind while you train.

Question:
Which is better: Curves or a regular gym?

Answer:
This is a difficult question because everyone is different. The typical gym has both men and women whereas Curves is a women's gym. The typical gym offers a variety of fitness classes, such as kickboxing, aerobics, yoga and spinning, as well as free weights and circuit training while Curves is a structured 30-minute program for circuit training.

Both are beneficial as long as you are working out. By working throughout your pregnancy, you will keep your muscles stronger/leaner and more viable which means a faster, healthier recovery after having the baby.

No matter where you go, be sure that the staff is properly certified and knowledgeable about pregnant clients. Be sure that your workouts are safe yet challenging. If you are bored, you will eventually quit.

At Home
Question:
I was just wondering if there is a fitness workout plan that I can follow to stay in shape during my pregnancy? I enjoy walking and lifting weights (3 lbs) to exercise my triceps and biceps. My significant other seems to think I need to work out in a gym in order to stay in shape. Can you please advise? Thanks.

Answer:
There is no need to go to the gym to get in shape. There are a variety of ways to work out to build muscle, endurance, flexibility -- all things you want to prepare yourself for labor.

Here are some tips to consider:

--All too often women work out to fight fat. Yes, yes, they know they are pregnant but remain hopeful they can stop the 'beached whale' image. This is not the time to be worried about appearance as much as you should want to prepare yourself for the 'big day' and post-partum days in caring for the baby.

--Many pregnant women who work out focus on one kind of work out. That is, some focus on lifting light weights because they have been told to stay away from 'impact' workouts. Others fear they will get 'bigger' by lifting weights and stick to more of a cardio program, such as walking, biking, or step. They best kind of workout includes both.

By lifting (light) weights, you build muscle. Even pregnant, a pound of muscle will burn four more calories a day than a pound of fat -- and yes, even pregnant, you can replace fat with muscle. It is possible to come out of a pregnancy in better shape than when you went in. By working with the nutritionists and trainer (who is qualified to work with pregnant clients), you can actually get into the best shape of your life.

Cardio is important because while it does burn fat -- not something we focus on at this point in your life/pregnancy -- this activity will prepare you for the endurance needed during labor & delivery. Many C-sections are the direct result of an exhausted mother who needs medical assistance when she can no longer push.

So, what can/should you do?
1) Check with your OB/GYN to get a green light for working out.
2) Contact a personal trainer. Many of my clients also work with a nutritionist at this time, keeping a food journal. You will be amazed how differently food affects your mood, energy, sleep, and complexion, not to mention weight.

It is difficult for give you a specific workout as I have very little information to go on. For example, if you only walk once or twice a week, at a leisurely pace, for about 15 minutes, I do not want to set you with a workout routine that exhausts you. All too often, women come to me in a panic because they just learned they are pregnant and suddenly want to work out. Wrong.

Continue with the exercise routine you are currently with.

Ideally, you want to work out four to five times a week. Take a look at this sample workout of a moderate workout:

Monday: Walk 2 mile
    Upper body workout: biceps, triceps, shoulders, lower back
    (there is a variety of workouts for each of these muscle groups. See

Part III)

Tuesday: Bike (stationary only!) -- 20 minutes
Walk if you do not have access to a stationary bike
Lower Body: extensions, hamstring, buttocks (leg press and squats)
(again, if you do not have access to a gym, there are a variety of
home exercises you trainer can provide)

Wednesday: Rest

Thursday Repeat of Monday with a variation of walking -- jog if possible
or change walking route

Friday: Repeat of Tuesday
Walk track with skip walking or lunges
*Bad knees? Skip the lunges and add an additional track lap or
¼ mile to your walk.

Saturday: Play exercise. This can a variety of activities that simply
raises your heart rate for swimming, basketball to hiking with a
friend.

4. Clothes: What to Wear

When it comes to clothing, women make two common mistakes in working out.
We spend so much time worrying about what matches, what *doesn't* make us look
fat, and what is in fashion that two vitals arc oftcn overlooked: shoes and bras.

Question:
*The size of my breasts have tended to fluctuate in the past, but now that I'm
pregnant they have gotten extremely large and heavy. I'm in my 7ᵗʰ month and
they feel weighed down. Is there anything I can do?*

Answer:
Yes, absolutely. What you wear and how you work out can help tremendously.
As your breasts get bigger (heavier), it begins to pull on your upper trapezius
(muscles running along behind your neck/shoulders). This can become increasing
painful and cause later back pains. By working out (working those specific
muscles and secondary supporting muscle groups),

you can alleviate those strains and build more muscle to support the breasts. But the kind of bra you wear can and will also help with support.

Many women do not exercise in their later months of pregnancy simply because of the bounce factor. Finding the right sports bra can minimize bouncing and make you feel more confident and secure.

Suggested bras for larger breasted women:

Brooks Pro-Support Bra, $52, sizes running from 32 to 40 D and 34 to42DD. It uses compression, encapsulation, and an underwire to reduce bounce. www.brooksrunning.com or (800) 227-6657

Moving Comfort Fiona Bra, $40, sizes 32C to 44DD. This is a great bra as the straps are "superadjustable" with a hook and loop strap that is perfect for anyone with shoulder and back problems. www.movingcomfort.com or (800) 763-6000.

A personal favorite is the Enell sports bra, tagged by Oprah as the ultimate sports bra. Self magazine stated, "Working out can really be painful if you're not wearing the right bra. For women with a D cup, their breasts can bounce more than 4-1/2 inches while they're jogging. From all that bouncing, your breast skin stretches, which leads to sagging over the long term. Hands down, this bra tested the best for motion control for larger sizes. Women with a larger-sized chest need substantial fabrics, straps that are at least 1 inch wide, a higher neckline, wider rib bands and a really sturdy cup. This bra really holds you in — you won't move at all!"

It is $51, sizes 32C to 52DD. (877) 567-5239.

If you are very busty, I highly recommend wearing two sports bras – doubling up – for the extra support. As we will discuss in 'pregnancy myths' damage to your breast tissue does not occur with breastfeeding but begins while you are pregnant. Now is the time to protect your breasts.

Shoes

Whether you are walking, jogging, taking step aerobics or working the circuit training program, it is important to have good shoes. As your body grows and shifts, as your weight increases, and your joints loosen, wearing quality shoes is imperative to overall good health.

In the running world, the general rule has always been to buy new shoes every 300 to 500 miles. But this counts only if the running shoes are used exclusively for running. If you are dusting off an old pair of shoes or simply wearing the same shoes you've had for six months, it's time to buy a quality shoe that offers shock absorption and proper cushioning for your foot.

If financially possible, own two pairs of athletic shoes: workout only and everyday walking around shoes. Your feet with thank you later.

5. Journaling

I know, I know. You're not one for journaling. But the purpose of journaling has tremendous benefits during your pregnancy. My own journaling began while training for the US bobsled team. As part of the research on pregnant athletes, it was important that I record what I ate, how I trained, how I felt during and after workouts, movements from the baby, and my sleep patterns. Initially, it was a royal pain in the rear end.

Then, I began to discover patterns in my workouts, able to predict when I was getting a cold or hadn't had enough sleep or water. By looking at my journal, I could see where I'd faltered nutritionally.

Beyond this, I was able to show how I'd been training to my physicians and my trainers who were with the bobsled program (not the research team). Finally, this is a journal that my daughter now cherishes as it is as much about her as it was my own training and dietary schedule.

Getting Started

Take a week to record your typical eating/drinking habits. Don't stress over exact amounts. If you eat two handfuls of M&Ms, simply write down "two handfuls." Be as honest and as accurate as you can, writing down glasses of water, sips of juice, cans of Coke. Record the times that you ate meals, what you had and where you were. For example, were you standing at the kitchen counter, watching t.v. when you ate a deli sandwich? Write these details down.

After one week of logging your meals, meet with a nutritionist. If you cannot afford this, there are many on-line organizations that have certified nutritionists who can analyze your journal.

This should be your first get-real look at how you eat and how committed you are to making healthy changes for you and the baby. Your commitment to keeping a detailed journal is your first step to a new lifestyle.

Taking Charge, Taking Notes

Once you've begun keeping a food journal, the next obvious step is to record your physical activity. This may come by working with a trainer or you may use examples presented in this book.

By keeping track of your work, you can no longer deny the truth. Over the years, I've had countless clients swear to me with all the sincerity they can muster, "I don't know why I'm gaining weight! I'm working out all the time!" As soon as we began to log how far they walked or biked, how long they worked out, how many bicep or leg curl repetitions they performed, however, they quickly realized how often they *thought* they worked out but never really did.

If you have three or four good workouts over a period of three weeks and you've always been a sedentary person, this may suddenly seem like a lot of physical activity. In truth, this is just one workout per week – not nearly enough to develop muscle, boost metabolism, or energize a person. These here-and-there workouts will only prolong soreness and stiffness, not something that will inspire a person to continue working out.

Even if you only walk a half-mile a day, write it down. This is something you can look back on, build on, and be proud of.

Baby Notes

Finally, imagine how much your baby will love the journal as he or she gets older. As your child reads how active he or she was, how you were kicked or kept awake, it is a personal joy for them. To this day, my children enjoy scrutinizing their varying tastes in food by what and how I ate. Example: Unfortunately for us all, my older child is well aware of the fact that I once ate an entire jar of Smuckers and believes this is why she isn't a big jelly fan.

6. Your Team

Olympic swimmer Angel Martino once said she approached her pregnancy as though she were in training for the Olympics – a different kind of Games. It was a healthy attitude that allowed her to remain positive rather than fear she was losing her edge in the water, gaining weight, or falling behind fellow swimmers in training. No surprise, she came back stronger than ever.

Although she was in an individual sport, she was part of a team during her pregnancy. You should approach your own pregnancy in this same manner. Team Baby should include your personal physician, OB/GYN, a trainer, a nutritionist, your significant other (if appropriate), a training buddy, and your journal. If you already have children, let them be part of Team Baby.

The Doctors

As discussed, it is important to work with your personal physicians. You must always get their medical permission to workout but beyond this, it is a great idea to keep them plugged into your training regimen, your trainers, and your long- and short-term goals.

You will be amazed how their interest and support will motivate you during your workouts and the way you eat. Knowing that your medical team is rooting for you, asking questions about your training when they see you, and noting the healthier you will give you even more incentive to get (or stay) fit.

The Trainer and Nutritionist

As part of Team Baby, you want to be sure these people are qualified. Like all good teams, teammates must have some connection to work well together. Do not feel pushed into working with a trainer or nutritionist if you don't like the person or feel awkward around him or her. I've heard numerous stories from women who worked with a male trainer and felt embarrassed or were intimidated by a "perfect" trainer or felt rushed during workouts as the trainer had other clients to work with. Right or wrong, the reality is if you're more focused on the trainer than what you are supposed to be doing, Team Baby has a problem.

Find a trainer who makes you feel comfortable, who takes the time to explain the purpose of different exercises and how each muscle group is being worked. Expect your trainer to know the latest training techniques, including the importance of inner core temperature, and do not be afraid to ask for (and call) references.

Don't know where to start looking for a nutritionist? Did you know that people who sell "health" products can call themselves "nutritional advisors" or "counselors", yet have no certification? You need to be wary of this. So, what is expert status?

The American Dietetic Association requires a four-year degree and a 9 to 12 month internship to qualify for the registered dietician (RD) credential, and candidates must pass a credited examination. Many RDs work in hospitals or other health-care facilities. To find a credited RD, log on to www.eatright.org.

A certified nutritionist must have a science or education in nutrition and take/pass an examination with the American Associations of Clinical Nutritionists (IAACN) to become an official CCN – certified clinical nutritionist. CCNs analyze how food affects you/your body and tailor a more suitable diet for your health and medical needs. To find a CCN near you, call (972) 407-9089.

Your Spouse or Significant Other

The role your spouse or significant other plays on Team Baby is invaluable. Consciously or unconsciously, more fitness programs and lifestyle changes have been sabotaged by nay-sayers and most often these nay-sayers are family. Because they are intimidated or inconvenienced by your sudden interest in something else, seemingly innocent comments such as, "You'll never be able to do that," or "Why are you doing that?" can become quite burdensome.

Let your significant other know how valuable they are to Team Baby. Include them in your goals, from fitness routines to grocery shopping. Most people have a habit they want to break or a goal they hope to achieve. Make this part of your new routine. Whether it's to run a 5k race or quite chewing tobacco, to start biking again or lose 15 pounds, mark down their goals with yours and work together. Isn't it only fair you're your family work for a goal along with yours?

Let them meet the rest of Team Baby. Often times, the nay-sayer will quickly change their tune when they hear everyone else singing praises.

Training Buddy

Studies show that women who workout together tend to stick with the fitness program longer, enjoy the exercise more, and have better results. When you are feeling particularly sluggish, your training buddy can motivate you to get up and get moving. Whether it's guilt, competition, or the simple desire to spend quality time with a friend, the training buddy is a key player in working out consistently.

But your training buddy is also valuable for safety reasons. Obviously, it is wise to walk or jog with a partner when you are outdoors but the training buddy can also help keep an eye on you while you are pregnant and training.

I like the buddy system as partners tend to notice when their buddy is breathing more heavily than normal, appears more labored or sweaty. Often times, the athletic mom-to-be may become so focused on 'finishing' the exercise, it takes a buddy to suggest, "Hey, you're breathing a little too hard. Why don't we walk a little," or "let's take a water break."

Your Journal

Your journal is very much a part of Team Baby. For this reason, you need to take the time to record in it just as you take time each day for specific chores or morning rituals, such as putting on make-up.

Other Children

Just as you should include your significant other in your training regimen, it's a great idea to include the other children in your life. In doing this, several things occur. They are empowered when you elicit their help. Dependent upon their age, they can help you journal and grocery shop.

Explain your goals, including no more fast food. Guess who wins with this goal? Everyone. Pediatricians are constantly trying to find ways to motivate American moms to stop the drive-thru habit. (See Chapter 11: I Want to Change My Eating Habits). While our children are being pumped full of preservatives, fillers, sugar, and unhealthy fats, you can break that trend. When your children believe they are part of an important program that will help you and baby, they will not disappoint. Children are amazing teammates.

Even toddlers can become part of Team Baby by stretching, walking, and joining a lifting program. Who says that while your lifting 4 or 5 lbs hand weights that your child cannot also lift soup cans, singing, "Yes, I can!"

One of the greatest gifts you can offer your children is the joy of working out. As they huff and puff next to you, earning your praise and attention, nothing could be better. And they will love to be included in your journal.

With Team Baby in play, let's talk about what is holding you back.

Chapter Two
Mirror, Mirror on the Wall

For Immediate Release
May 5, 2005

"Pregnancy.org – "I'm a 33-year-old, non-motivated, married-with-children female," writes Cathy in her online fitness journal. "I've gained weight. I've lost weight. I've gained it back again. I've lost it again. It's time to be accountable ... and to be a healthy role model for my children."

Cathy is one of 12 women worldwide chosen to participate in Alexandra Powe Allred's online fitness makeover, sponsored by the mega-parenting website www.pregnancy.org.

"Pregnancy has historically been seen as a time of "confinement' or inactivity," says Allred. "In fact, the key is to be active, eat right, and stay healthy before, during and beyond pregnancy."

"Allred understands what woman are facing when they want to make major lifestyle changes," says pregnancy.org's founder and owner, Mollee Olenick. "America's obesity crisis is fueled by our time crunch. Finding time for the gym or a personal trainer is next to impossible for today's busy families."

Once again the parenting website has found innovative ways to use the power of the Internet to help families. The "Determined Dozen" won't be meeting in a gym, but they will keep online eating journals, meet strict exercise goals, and report to Allred by phone and e-mail once a week. On-line meetings using pregnancy.org's chat software will provide encouragement and keep the women accountable to each other for exercise and diet commitments.

The Determined Dozen were fun because they represented every woman. Tall, short, thin, overweight, medical problems, perfect health, single, married, first-time moms to a mother of eight children. While one battled with smoking issues, another dealt with eating disorders. Some loved to exercise, others had never broken a sweat. We had vegetarians and junk-food junkies, Starbuck-aholics and those who looked at water as something to be dreaded. I've also worked with elite athletes, professional models, fitness experts, and hard-core exercisers who could not fathom the idea of backing away from athletics while pregnant.

However diverse the groups, all of these women shared common concerns about weight gain, how the scale might read, appearance, overall health and, of course, having a healthy baby.

"For women who want to lose weight! Keep on bearing children as long and often as possible."

- Creative and Sexual Science, 1876

1. Body Image

"I know I should be so happy. I've wanted to be pregnant for so long and now all I can think about is how fat I am getting. Help!"

<u>Answer</u>:

Believe it or not, this is a common feeling. Don't beat yourself up. The worry of gaining too much weight and what others may think of you is a common mommy-to-be worry. There are some very positive things you can focus on while pregnant that will carry over into the way you see yourself, the way you want to train and eat. More importantly, it will give you a healthier, happier attitude about that precious baby to come.

1. Your Baby: The world sees and comments about *you* to you. For that reason, it is very easy to get caught up in you, you, you. Re-channel that energy. Marvel in the miracle of birth. Be in awe that as you sit reading this book, a baby is growing inside of you. Be humbled by how amazing women are and what wonderful things your body is doing to create this life.

2. Your Health: With that, ask yourself, "What can I do to help?" Be sure to take your prenatal vitamins, drink enough water, stay away from junk foods and colas. Take pride in that your healthy lifestyle and your dedication to living more healthily is a tribute to your baby.

3. Ignore the Mirror on the Wall: Focus on what is really important. Your current image is only a temporary one. Do not focus on your weight or the image in the mirror. Instead, remember this is all part of a process. You will gain weight, you will say goodbye to your feet (temporarily), you may have acne break outs or become bloated. Despite how you may feel by the ninth month – this really is only temporary.

4. Use Your Mother Voice: Congratulations. Not long from now, you are going to give birth to someone who will eventually not listen to you, forget what you've told them, repeatedly misunderstand what you say, and unintentionally hurt your feelings. You may as well start practicing your mother voice now! The next time someone hurts your feelings or says something critical about you/your growing form, speak up and let them know how you feel.

5. Ignore Media Role Models: What? Supermodels posing in bikini-impregnated form? Puh-lease! Look, what matters is your health. Are you working out? Eating and resting well?

Question:

I feel like a cave woman! My hormones are going crazy and I'm hungry all the time. How am I supposed to watch my weight if all I can do is think about eating?

Answer:

You are a cave woman. How do you like that?

Ever notice how easily men can lose weight? It seems that no sooner do they announce they are going to lose weight, it's off. It is maddening for those of us who have to sweat and starve just to make a dent on the "bathroom scale diet." Typical of so many men, my husband tells stories of his days as an All-State high school wrestler. He would starve himself for days before the weigh-in to ensure he competed in his desired weight class, then gorge himself to increase his weight come the wrestling match. It seems that wrestlers and boxers do this all the time. He'll also tell me he has days at work when he's "forgotten" to eat. I don't understand this. I lie in bed at night thinking about what I will have for breakfast the next morning and often plan my lunch menu while eating breakfast. How can you forget to eat?

But I've been working on a theory for years now and believe I'm right. It all goes back to the time of hunters and gatherers. Listen up because how well you grasp and embrace this concept may determine your success in developing and sculpting your body in the manner that pleases you. Early in our life together, I began to make note of my husband's behavior. No matter how you dress them up, no matter how nicely you try to decorate and turn the cave into a homey dwelling, men will always be cavemen. Oh, sure, you can take the man out of the cave . . . You know how that goes. This is why men can 'forget' to eat. Many a moon would pass and early man would travel great distances before seeing a mammoth to kill and feed upon. It's why men don't really like to talk too much. You can't track mammoth while gabbing away on the hunter trail. And, it's why modern man has greater muscle mass than women. They had to do the whole, "Argh! Mad mammoth at six o'clock" sprint thing to survive out there in the wilds. Women, on the other hand, never had our nuts and berries turn on us, and we never had to wrestle an herb to the ground. Women, a.k.a. 'the gatherers' munched throughout the day. We talked to one another, watched the kids, and collected those berries and nuts in our baskets. "One berry for the community basket and one berry for me." We'd pop some in our mouths and continue to talk about our stupid cavemen. "One nut for the community basket and one nut for me." Pop. We were stuck at the cave, listening to old lady Unga Unga talking about her old caveman, and all of his weird habits, while dozens of wild cave children ran around us screaming. By God, we needed those extra nuts and berries.

Throughout history, until modern times, this was the life of the female. It wasn't until the last several decades that women have seriously gotten into the hunter role. But what with millions of years of genetic makeup dictating otherwise, it is hard to convince our bodies that we no longer need to eat like gatherers. No wonder losing fat seems especially hard for women and that keeping it off is a constant battle. No sooner do we begin to lose weight than our bodies release hormones signaling to the body it is hungry and needs to be replenished.

As a self-protective measure, your metabolism – the fat burner -- slows down to ensure you don't lose too much weight too quickly. Of course, that quick weight loss is what we most desire, but we are dealing with evolution in reverse. Our bodies aren't entirely convinced that we haven't run out of nuts and berries; they want to be sure that we make it through the harsh winter – even if we are living in Florida.

And therein lies the problem. History dictates that our bodies should be gatherers – social, nut-collecting fat-storers while men remain uncommunicative, wandering fat-burners. Women (and modern men) find temporary success on diets that are similar to the early hunters': High protein, low carbs, eating huge portions until satisfied but only a few times a day with intermittent bursts of physical activity follows the regimen of many modern-day Akins dieters today. But after a time, most of us go back to the modern conveniences of fast food and remote controls, allowing sedentary lives and super-sized food portions to again become the norm. (Believe me, one of the problems cavemen had was not getting enough fat and there was never any threat of consuming too much glucose.)

But before you get too excited about the lifestyle of the early cave people, remember this: They lived very short lives. Besides the very real possibility of being eaten by a saber-tooth tiger, they died of malnutrition, dehydration, and disease. Most never had the displeasure of experiencing osteoporosis because of all the other fatality factors; however, for the few who made it past 40 years of age, brittle, calcium-deprived bones were a painful reality according to paleontologists.

Today there are so many dicts on thc markct, so many promises, so many 'fat-burners', so many exercise gimmicks and so many, many failed dieters one has to wonder if anyone really has the answer. Well, my fellow former cave-dwelling, fat-storing gatherers, the answer is 'yes.' The answer did not come to me until I was in my most natural, most maternal state. Flat stomachs look nice but there is a reason we have hips, store fat, and have breasts. Once you have a realistic and appreciative understanding of why we are built the way we are, you won't feel quite so critical of yourself. Still, this enlightenment is not a license to sit on the couch all day eating Big Macs.

Our cave-dwelling ancestors didn't get lean by sitting around the campfire, getting themselves wired on 'fat burning' pills. They worked. They ate healthy (non-fried) carbs and meats. They weren't looking for an overnight change. Neither should we. And, I assure you, when they were pregnant, they did not obsess over weight gain. Weight gain for the cavewoman as a good thing!

Now that you are pregnant, think like a cavewoman. Stop kidding yourself. Be prepared to eat well. No junk food. Be prepared to make exercise a way of life. Be prepared to do some form of cardio for 30 to 45 minutes, four times a week. Lift weight using lower weights and higher repetitions to create lean muscle mass.

Alternate your upper and lower body workouts, allowing your muscles to rest properly before the next training session. For those of you who really and truly cannot make it to a gym, train at home four times a week, lift weights twice a week, working the overall body. Be sure to give your body at least two days of recovery before lifting again. Include interval training. Whether you ride a stationary bike or simply walk the track, give yourself an hour a week to increase your metabolism and work new muscle groups. This kind of training will dramatically increase your fitness level. When you are no longer pregnant, this will be the beginning of your weight loss/control regiment. Don't forget to stretch. Long, lean, healthy muscles come from stretching. As you stretch more and more, you will increase flexibility, which will help your balance, reduce muscle injuries, and build range of motion.

Finally, forget everything you ever heard about "no pain, no gain." Yes, yes, it is supposed to be challenging when you lift weights, ride the bike, and jog laps. It should be hard, you should be sweating but it should never be painful to the point of injury. I always tell my kickbox classes, unless there is a multi-million dollar contract on the line, millions of adoring fans and photographers ready to capture your every move... why would you willing to hurt yourself? Trust me, there is no glory in the emergency room when you are sitting all alone next to some guy hacking up a lung. If it's challenging – wonderful. If it hurts, stop.

Dedicate yourself to a new you. Water, proper nutrition, a safe workout routine, and a goal. As you log in your journal, write down the number of reps, times, and steps into your own personal fitness book. You will be amazed how you progress, how quickly time flies, and how much stronger you feel. Most importantly, find something you can have fun with. It has been my experience that training with a buddy helps keep you on track. It is possible for you to be a hunter and a gatherer.

Embrace the new cave you.

2. The Scale
Question:
I recently purchased a Homedics scale with the body fat analysis feature. I'm 34 years old, about 5'3 and weigh around 100 lbs. I am pretty active and lean, but the body fat analysis showed me that I had 28% body fat on the first day and then up to 34% the next day. I was mortified and concerned because I am very body and weight conscious. The instructions stated that the body fat analysis is not for children, pregnant women, or athletes. Why is this? Why would my body fat register so much higher? I was just 18% body fat a few years ago at the same weight."

Answer:
Akkk!
Don't look at that again. And I will tell you why .. they are not always reliable and because, as you say, you are very body and weight conscious, it will only drive

you crazy with worry. Although there are now a number of popular ways to calculate body fat, they cannot properly tabulate the weight of your bone and muscle mass as oppose to how much of your weight is actually fat. Water retention, recent salt-intake, day-to-day fluctuation, your menstrual cycle, and even the time of day can alter results. The absolute best way to learn your true body fat count is hydrodensitomerty weighing or underwater weighing. This procedure, while certainly more expensive, can accurately determine bone, muscle, and fat content.

Unless you are an elite athlete or a competitive bodybuilder, this really should not matter. How you feel and regular physicals with your doctor should be most important. But there are a few other things to consider. It is important to understand that you will naturally begin to lose some muscle mass now that you've entered the 30s. Just because a person has only 18% body fat – very good, by the way – in their 20s doesn't mean things will stay the same even if you keep the same diet/fitness routine. When you are not pregnant, this is a good reason to meet with a trainer and find a new routine – mix things up a little and challenge your body/muscles.

Please remember that it is really the scale that is unpredictable, not you.

Having said this, however, a pregnant woman does not need to be looking at her fat content. Leave that to your doctor.

Recently, I worked with a client who is very conscious about her weight, size, and fat. As a result, she ate very little in her second pregnancy, had an unhealthy approach to her growing belly and had a baby under five lbs at full term. Knowing this, she still struggles with diet and body image in her third pregnancy. At this point, there are some very important things to focus on. Exercise. Water. Proper diet. Rest. And proper body image.

You can keep the same exercise routine, altering slightly as you move through the trimesters. I strongly recommend that you work with a personal trainer from time to time to be sure your movement and weights are safe for you/baby. But you can stay strong and keep your metabolism active so that you will be able to recover all the more quickly after your baby is born.

Stay hydrated and speak to a nutritionist about your current diet. Perhaps you are eating more saturated fats than you think. For example, if you are eating frozen, precooked meals, even if it calls itself a "lean" meal, you may not be eating as healthy as you've been lead to believe. This could explain the sudden (unlikely) fat count change.

Lastly, is rest. This cannot be overstated. While I worry half my clients are too sedentary, there is that other side who think because they are pregnant they *can't* sit still. But proper rest is just as important as working out.

The most important thing you can do is put that scale away! Away! Away, I say!

Let your doctor know that you tend to worry about your weight and talk about why that is. Are you worried about 'getting fat' and staying that way? Or, do you have a family history of obesity and health related issues? Are you determined to stay in a certain clothing size? Do you have a sister or mother-in-law who consistently points out your weight gain to you? Talk to your OB/GYN about these very real and important feelings and make a pact that s/he will watch and monitor your weight for you. The first sign of a problem, you will have a sit down with a personal trainer or nutritionist. Otherwise, no worries, no weighing, no judging!!

I've worked with a number of elite athletes who obsessed over their body weight while pregnant because they were acutely aware of how hard it would be to get back to Olympic form if they gained too much weight. Every woman later said she wished for her baby's sake that she had relaxed and just let nature take its course. Think of growing your baby like an Olympic event. It doesn't happen overnight and neither does getting back into shape – but that really is a good thing as you develop new (good) habits, discover new and exciting ways to train and develop better muscle groups as you get back into shape after having your baby. Flo-Jo, Marion Jones, Peggy Fleming, Mary Lou Retton, Joy Fawcett, Gabrielle Reece, Linda Hanley, Sheryl Swoopes, and Gwen Torrence (to name a few Olympic athletes) all have said that they were in better, faster, stronger, and healthier AFTER having a baby.

Let that be your motto!

Good luck and enjoy your pregnancy.

3. Obesity

Primarily, these questions come from Northern American residents. But the number of obesity related questions regarding pregnancy, health, and fitness seems to be increasing. My honest response to this is: Great! I'm pleased that overweight and/or clinically obese women are taking a hard and serious look at their current situation.

Here is a sampling of the kind of questions I receive:

"How overweight is too overweight to be pregnant? Is it dangerous to the baby to be obese? I'm 23 and at least 100 lbs. overweight and would like to become pregnant within the next year. Advice?"

"I'm 150-pounds overweight. I eat pretty good, don't drink colas but I can't stand water. I drink a lot of juice and ice tea and would like to start an exercise and diet regiment, but I'm at a loss as to where to get started. Any suggestions? I wanna be a healthy mom, but I have absolutely no clue how to do that."

"I'm 5'2" and weight 215 lbs. I'm pretty active but don't eat so good. I was wondering what are my chances for carrying a healthy baby? I know that the ideal weight gain is 25-30 pounds. What suggestions can you give me so I only gain what I need to? And what is the least amount of weight I can gain and still be healthy?"

"I am having my third child. I am trying to get healthy as well. I am 5'8" and weight 235 lbs. We have diabetes in my family and I am worried about my weight during pregnancy. Any advice?"

Answers to these questions tend to sound simplistic, even condescending. Talk to your doctor, see a trainer and nutritionist about beginning a safe exercise routine and better eating habits.

Oh, gee! Okay. Let me get right on that and drop a hundred pounds.

It's not that easy. You know it. I know it.

But the fact that you are asking questions, are seeking better health, and are concerned for the future of your baby are all great indicators that you want to be a healthier, happier person, that you want to take the role of mother seriously, and that you have a chance of great success.

The reality is this: The heavier you are, the more difficult it is going to be to find energy, ignore outside factors such as comments, poor self-esteem and personal motivation. The heavier you are, the more difficult it is going to be to actually move. The strain is difficult on your joints. The heavier you are, the more difficult it can be to conceive.

You must first speak to your doctor because of the likelihood of diabetes, high blood pressure, and heart disease, to name a few. These medical conditions become even more serious when pregnant. For these reasons, you must speak with your doctor before starting any kind of physical routine. The hard realities are that with significantly overweight women who conceive are at greater risk of giving birth to babies with birth defects. For this reason, doctors strongly urge that women get into better physical condition before getting pregnant.

Having said this, however, there are plenty of overweight to obese women who have had perfectly healthy pregnancies and babies. Is this my permission then to be or stay out of shape? Absolutely not! But if you are already pregnant and are very overweight to obese, I want you to feel that you can still take control of this situation. There is no reason to obsess or stress over your current physical condition.

At this precise moment, be proud of yourself for picking up this book, thinking about the futures for both you and your baby. I offer you the same advice I give my elite athletes. The weight didn't come on overnight and it's not going to leave anytime soon. Your weight, your pregnancy, your attitudes, your lifestyle changes – all gradual processes. The beauty of this, then, is that you can begin making small changes today. Nothing radical, so don't panic.

1. Stop drinking sodas. Even diet. I know, I know… you will curl up and die without your daily soda(s). But by eliminating soda pop from your diet, you will lose between 20-26 pounds within a year without even changing anything else in your life. Because these drinks are so addictive, it may be a struggle. Studies show that soda pop drinkers are more

2. addicted to sugars and tend to eat more sugary/fatty snacks throughout the day. A recent study had one group of people eat jelly beans (solid calories) and another group consume an equal amounts of calories from soda pop (liquid calories). The jelly bean group ultimately consumed less calories throughout the day whereas the liquid group did not feel satisfied and continued to snack.

3. More water. Simply put, when you drink more water and replace your sugary drinks (this includes juices) with water, you will drop weight. If pregnant, this will also help you reduce bloating, decrease morning sickness, and cleanse toxins from your body.

4. Hello, grill! In Chapter Three, you will read about our relationship to food. I hope this will help you better understand the benefits and pitfalls of eating. That is, how, when, and where you eat. And, of course, why. But while you're busily gnawing on that, introduce yourself to the grill. Whether you live in an apartment (use the balcony) or purchase the George Foreman grill for your kitchen, grilling meats and veggies offer some great eating habits.

   A.) Learn to wait. The need for instant gratification when it comes to food is a dangerous habit for us all. Learning to prepare foods rather than pulling into a drive-thru is the greatest weapon against poor eating habits!

   B.) You can break the 'fried food' cycle!

   C.) Your taste buds will change. If you love food – I mean, really love food – you know that fried and fatty foods lack the true taste. Grilled chicken, grilled veggies are bursting with the true flavor Mother Nature intended. Here is a chilling fact: The true junk food junkie will turn her nose up at the grill because her taste buds have been so compromised by grease and preservatives. If this is you, be sure to read Chapter Three. Rent the movie, **SuperSize Me**. Educate yourself on what it is you are really eating.

5. Begin a routine. Again, you must get medical permission before starting any kind of exercise routine. But once you've been given the green light, start up and don't look back. Whether you begin swimming, pool aerobics, or walking, give yourself realistic goals. You will find sample exercise routines in Part III of this book. But I strongly urge that you meet with a trainer – even just once – to assess your physical conditioning and determine what is safe for you to do. Find a training buddy and begin.

6. Define "Fit!" Get the image of a super buff Demi Moore or svelt Angelina Joli out of your head. You can be overweight and in shape. In truth, 60-, 80, 100+ pounds are too much but you also don't have to be a size 8 to look and feel great. Trust me when I tell you, I've conducted many a kickbox class where the skinny girl ran outside to throw up while the bigger gals punched and kicked the hour away!

Question:

"I need help. I have been married 5 years and since the day my husband and I got married we stopped using protection so we can get pregnant. After a year of trying we went to see my doctor. I was not getting a monthly period so he started me on Provera and Clomid due to irregular periods. I started both medications but was not getting pregnant. The doctor said it is most likely of my weigh, at the time I was 442 pounds, that was in 2002. I decided to lose weight and weighed 343 pounds last April (four years later). After a series of medications [to get pregnant] I noticed the pills made me lazy and so tired that I even stopped working out. Needless to say, I gained all my weight back and now weigh 437 and back to square one. We just found out that my husband's insurance covers the treatment [fertility] and we want to start this summer, but now I am scared because of my weight, scared the doctor might turn us down. I had started slowly doing the treadmill and plan to do it every day and watch what I am eating, all I want now is to be a mother and have a baby. I need advice. Can I still get pregnant when I am obese? Do you know anyone who weighed as much as I did and got pregnant and everything is fine with the baby?"

Answer:

Do not despair. There are things you can do and I am pleased to hear that you are concerned about your weight and ready to do something about it. As a mother, you want to be two things, 1) a role model and, of course, 2) healthy so that you can be an active mom. So, with that, let's talk strategy.

You always hear stories about women gaining weight during pregnancy. This is Mother Nature's way of preparing the body and baby for healthy growth and delivery. But for women who are already heavy, the weight gain is not necessary and, remarkably, your body knows this. We can devise plans that will enable you to carry a healthy baby to full term with minimal gain. But first … You MUST talk to your doctor. Before you begin any exercise – even your treadmill – get medical permission. Lay out your goals in terms of weight, future pregnancy hopes, medications, and your current physical condition.

Next, you need to make an appointment with a nutritionist. Because of your medical condition (obesity), there may also be a chance that your insurance will pay for you to see a nutritionist. Check into this possibility.

We've discussed Team Baby before and will set you on course to develop this helpful team but you have another worry: worry. Negative thoughts, stress over conception can actually interfere with getting pregnant. No surprise, once you begin working out and eating better, stress naturally decreases. As you begin to feel better both emotionally and physically, it is amazing how your body will respond.

Last year, a group of women who worked out, logged on-line to discuss their frustrations, setbacks, successes, and worries. It was a great success and so many were surprised by their will power and strength, but all noted that having a support group was most inspiring.

As you begin to eat and train for a healthier lifestyle, remember those very powerful words you spoke: "I want to be a mother." If you really mean that, you can do this. That feeling alone will empower you but Team Baby is vital. Get friends and family on board, and make sure your husband is ready for this commitment.

Okay, so you're over 400 pounds. Yes, you have your work cut out for you but you can do this.
1. Doctor.
2. Trainer
3. Nutritionist
4. Friends/Family
5. On-Line support group

Once you've come to terms with these very simple and lifesaving concepts, you really can take control of your pregnancy. Over the years, this is a recurring theme I've both espoused and heard. "Taking control."

An ideal weight gain does not necessarily apply when you are both pregnant and overweight. Again, this is why you need to let your doctors look at the scale. I have worked with women who gained only a few pounds throughout their entire pregnancy and others who packed on 80 lbs. It depends on the woman, her body, genetics, her lifestyle.

When Lili McCutchan, an at-home mom, went into her pregnancy, she was determined to "take control." While McCuthan was certainly not obese, she was conscious of her weight at 164 pounds at 5'6". Having never worked out, she got her doctors permission and began working with a professional trainer and dietician throughout her pregnancy. Following the birth of her daughter, McCuthan actually came out of her pregnancy at 161 pounds and in the best shape of her life.

If you eat well, cut out the liquid candy (colas, diet colas, fruit juices, Starbucks …), get with a walking program, and work with a trainer and/or training buddy, you will be amazed how strong you will feel.

4. **Underweight**
"Hi. I have a question. I am 26 years old and weigh about 95 pounds. We are thinking about having a baby soon, but I need to work on gaining weight. Please advise how I could achieve this."

"I'm planning to get pregnancy next year and heard that being underweight or having low body fat can make it more difficult. I'd like to stay active and have a good fitness routine but I lose body fat very fast when I exercise. I'm 5'2" and am just under 100 pounds. I eat a healthy 3 meals a day, snack 2-3 times a day. Should I be doing something different to try to gain more body fat before I attempt pregnancy? Is there exercise you can recommend that would keep me from losing my body fat too quickly?"

While the general thinking is the lower the body fat, the harder it is to conceive, Olympic athletes and marathon runners get pregnant all the time. Beyond lower body fat, there are other factors involved such a diet and inner core temperature (See Chapters Three and Four). Like the overweight mother-to-be, studies have shown that the chances of having a premature baby increases significantly with an underweight mother. According to the National Academy of Sciences, underweight women should gain a minimum of 28 to 40 pounds by 40 weeks.

If you are a highly active person, for example, running eight to 10 miles a day, heat can be a huge factor for both getting pregnant and gaining weight. As you run or aerobicize, your inner core temperature gets higher and higher. It has been argued that this makes conception more difficult and more researchers believe that elite athletes will abort without ever knowing they were ever pregnant due to intense training. Remember, however, these elite athletes are so singly focused on better split times, more grueling routes, higher jumps, and heavier weights that they may not even be thinking about pregnancy (or safety). But for the recreational athlete, you can remain more focused on better nutrition, hydration, and rest.

By working with a professional trainer to assess your physical conditioning, the two of you can discuss your goals: pregnancy, ideal weight, and workout program. Working hand-in-hand with a nutritionist, you can create (and keep) a food journal that will help you gain or maintain a specific weight. You may find that in your quest to get pregnant or continue a healthy weight during pregnancy, your intense running routine may have to be sidelined for a different kind of lower-calorie burning exercise.

Because you are underweight, you may also be in store for another change: instant weight gain. Women who are underweight will sometimes have a sudden weight gain when they first become pregnant. This condition – known as Mother Fuel – is often a surprise to new moms, as they fear this is a precursor to continued weight gain.

As you read the story of Olympian Michelle Rohl in initial weight gain (Mother Fuel), you will learn that how you react to this initial weight gain is important to both you and baby. Again, knowledge is power.

Having said all of this, of course, you must see your doctor. It is important that your personal physician – your team – is on board with the trainer and nutritionist.

The Underweight Couch Potato

But what if you are underweight and don't even exercise? While others repeatedly tell you how "lucky" you are, you know the other side of the coin and it isn't all gloss and shine.

You may have a built-in furnace that just seems to burn calories no matter what you do. You may have little to no appetite, an eating disorder, and a medical condition that prevents you from weight gain.

Your first step is an obvious one. You must make an appointment to see your personal physician and OB/GYN. Have a serious, honest, open conversation about your concerns and what it is you want. Weight gain, for the most part, can be relatively easy with the proper diet and exercise routine. But, again, everyone must be on board for Team Baby. You will need to keep a journal on your activities, diet, and exercise routine. This journal should be open to your teammates – the trainer, nutritionist, and medical staff – to evaluate and periodically change or update.

Let me give you an example of being honest and what is needed:

I received an e-mail from overseas from a woman who wanted reassurances that she could continue to hike while pregnant. The open response to this was if it is a sport or activity that you have been doing for some time, in which your muscles and cardio are completely acclimated to and you have medical permission, there should be no reason to stop. Of course, with this came the lecture on proper hydration, inner core temperature, hiking with a buddy, heart rate, and so on.

The following day, I received a 'thank you' for the information and permission to continue. I had had a sense that there was more to the story than I'd been told. I sent back a note with a few more questions regarding her current medical condition. It was then that I learned that she was considered a "high risk" by her doctor, who had discouraged her from hiking high altitudes.

Hmmm.

Oh, yes, and she was pregnant with triplets.

Oh, yes, and she was 5'10" and 120 pounds.

Akkk!

Red flags were popping up everywhere.

I sent yet another note to request a log of her everyday eating habits.

One look at her food journal and I knew that we had a serious problem. No protein, almost no complex carbohydrates. Too little fat.

Oh, yes, I have had an eating disorder in the past.

She was at more "high risk" than even she realized. While she was genuinely thrilled to be pregnant – and had been trying to get pregnant for some time – and recognized that she was medically underweight, she was also overly concerned about gaining "fat" weight. Without realizing it, she had not been honest about her present condition and was simply looking for someone to tell her it was okay to hike – alone – for long periods of time, with triplets, on a virtually empty stomach as a "high risk" candidate.

Again, if you are just a calorie-burning machine, your weight issue can safely be monitored and adjusted with the help of professionals. As you work out and build muscle, you will feel so much stronger, healthier, and happier. I promise.

But if you are clinically underweight for other reasons, let's find out why. I promise that if you build a strong Team Baby team, including your doctors, a trainer, a nutritionist, a training buddy, and family, not only will you become stronger physically but your self-esteem will sky-rocket.

Be honest to yourself and to Team Baby for baby.

5. Eating for Two

You are not eating for two. You are eating for you. That's the simple answer. However, it's more complicated than that because, in effect, you are what you eat. The better nourished and hydrated you are, the better it is for your baby. But the plain truth of it is, your baby takes whatever he or she needs from your body, often leaving the momma feeling depleted and fatigued.

The newly pregnant mom then decides on one definite thing: I should eat more!

"I am 27 years old and am pregnant. I gained as much as much 4 kilograms (8.8 pounds) in one month. How much should my weight increase in one month?"

"I haul heavy boxes at work all day long. Now I just found out I am pregnant. How should I eat now? How many calories should I eat?"

"I have been training with my sister to run a race for Breast Cancer and I just found out I'm pregnant. My doctor says I can go ahead and run the race but what should I eat while I am in training. Half the time I feel sick and the other half of the time, I am starving. But I don't want to gain a bunch of weight."

"I have been doing water aerobics and have lost a lot of weight!! Now I am pregnant and am afraid it is all going to come back. Can you give me a good diet?"

How's this for some helpful advice? I refuse! In Chapter Four, I discuss the healthful benefits and pitfalls of foods, things to think about and how to shop at the grocery store but there is no way I could possibly offer a 'diet' for a pregnant woman – active or sedentary. Too many factors are involved. And I want you to be wary of any on-line advice or diets that do not take your medical history, exercise routine, age, physique, and personal history into account before spitting out a mainstream diet.

1. Make an appointment with your OB/GYN
2. Begin your journal: both food and everyday activities. If you walk to the post office every morning at 8 a.m., write that down. If you sneak off to McDonald's when no one is looking, write that down.
3. Make an appointment – after one full week of keeping an honest journal – with a nutritionist. If you cannot afford to see this person more than once, don't be shy about this. Tell him or her, "Look, I just found out I'm pregnant. I've been keeping a journal on how I eat and workout and would like to come in, talk to you and have you look at what I'm doing." Together, you can take a critical look at how you are doing – you may be pleasantly surprised – and write out some long-term goals for your pregnancy.

This is absolutely the best way to determine what and how you should be eating while pregnant as it applies to your particular lifestyle. It drives me crazy when "full proof" diets are published with little regard to a person's medical and personal background.

Are you eating for two? No. But are you focused on what is best for your baby? Absolutely.

"I am two weeks pregnant and I am wondering if it is normal for a woman to lose a couple of pounds in the beginning or should I speak with my OB. Thank you, concerned new mom."

Don't panic. This happens quite often. However, it is always a good idea to talk to your OB/GYN, get a check-up and discuss how/what you are eating, your current weight and medical history. I do not believe in weighing in at the doctors unless one suffers from diabetes or other medical conditions where weight gain or loss has to be factored in. But when you are pregnant, it is a good idea to let your OB/GYN – another reason to keep regular appointments – keep an eye on rapid weight gain or loss.

Having said this, many women (particularly more active women) will initially lose a little weight and think, "Oh, hey! I'm losing weight! Isn't this great?" only to discover they are pregnant. If the weight loss totals more than ten pounds, do call in for an appointment. Otherwise, enjoy the brief reprieve. It's going to come back.

"How can I be gaining weight so fast?? I'm barely eating! What will happen to me if I keep gaining this much weight throughout my entire pregnancy? I'll weight 400 lbs.!"

This is exactly why I don't like fixed numbers. We can't possibly tell pregnant women how much weight they can and should gain or how many calories they should consume when everyone is different. While one woman may initially lose weight, others may pack on instant weight. And as common as it is to lose, it is equally common to suddenly find ten pounds in the first trimester.

6. Initial Weight Gain: Mother Fuel

"I gained ten pounds in the first month of my pregnancy," says Michelle Rohl, a former All-American distance runner and Olympic racewalker. "Now I know it is normal for my body. Since my percent of body fat is normally very low, my body knows it needs to store enough fat to support my pregnancy as quickly as possible. I didn't understand this yet. I thought, "If I keep gaining ten pounds a month, I will gain 90 pounds by the end of the pregnancy!"

During her first pregnancy, Rohl was determined that this pregnancy would not slow her down and she promised herself she would continue to train no matter what. But, she says, "Reality soon set in. While some people can continue for several months into their pregnancy without seeing a detriment in their training and racing, I am not one of those people. I tend to slow down significantly in the first two months, and then level off."

But having no previous experience with pregnancy, Rohl began to worry about her performance, fearing that if she was already slowing in her first trimester, she would be doubly slow in the third trimester. Comparing herself to other pregnant athletes she had known, Rohl feared she would never get back into shape.

It was fall when Rohl got pregnant with her daughter, Molly, so she decided to run with the University of Wisconsin-Parkside cross-country team. Rohl now reflects, "I wouldn't recommend this." It's only depressing to run the same workouts, with the same people week in and week out, watching yourself get slower and slower as more people begin to blow past you with each workout."

Still, Rohl was present for every race, never giving way to her growing belly and changing body. "[My] coach stopped giving me goal passes. He didn't want to be party to my obsession, but I was still obsessed with the stopwatch and my position in races and even workouts. I also began to have an unhealthy attitude toward my diet. I never really worried about diet or weight loss before I was pregnant; I ate whatever I wanted to eat."

Racewalking is an event that burns many calories, and Rohl had always eaten enough to support her training, but the weight gain was a concern.

Although this initial weight (called Mother Fuel by experts) is very healthy Rohl says she fixated on her weight, constantly stepping on the scale, making sure she didn't gain more than four pounds a month after that first month. In the end, Rohl only put on 20 pounds, and she believes that the one positive thing that came from all her worrying was becoming a better, healthier eater. But her attitude about workouts and weight gains were not healthy.

Rohl continued to train throughout her entire pregnancy. "My due date was July 18th, but I didn't believe this. I gained so much weight so early that I was sure I had to have conceived earlier. Therefore, I decided that the Fourth of July would be a good day to have the baby. This was a particularly hot day for Wisconsin, I remember, I went to the track. 'Eight hard quarters should put me into labor,' I thought. Ninety-second quarters were never so hard. Luckily, I came to my senses after four." With a pulse rate of 200 beats per minute, her face bright red, and calves so cramped that she was on her knees as she gasped for breath, Rohl decided the baby wasn't coming and limped back to the car.

She took it easy for the next few days running light one- or two-mile jogs. Molly arrived on July 7th. "I felt so sorry and guilty when I saw her. The doctor said she decided she was wrong about the due date, in the other direction. Instead of being one to one and half weeks early, she was three weeks early. Molly [baby] just looked like she'd rather crawl back inside and bake a little longer, and I wished I could accommodate her. While she was inside of me sometimes she seemed to be little more than a growing tumor that made me fat and slowed down my workouts. Now, she was a tiny, fragile, precious little girl. Being the best athlete suddenly plummeted on my list of priorities in life. I just wanted to be Molly's mother."

Since that time, Rohl went on to represent the United States in the 1992 and 1996 Olympic Games and, set an American record at the Goodwill Games. But what Rohl is most satisfied with is what she learned during her pregnancies and the joy her children have brought her. "I feel so lucky to have had the opportunity to do everything I've done in my life so far. Sometimes people say about me, 'Think of how good she would have been if she hadn't taken time out to have babies.' Maybe. But I wouldn't trade what I have for all the gold medals in the world!'"

7. **Your Team**

Had Michelle Rohl had a Team Baby and had she known what we now know about Mother Fuel, her experience would have been so much better. Had she had a training partner to reign her in, a trainer to analyze her workouts, or even a journal to look at her eating habits, she most certainly would have had more peace of mind and the confidence that everything was okay.

The role of your team, the communication you have with your training buddy, family members, doctors, and trainers is invaluable. Make the most of it.

Chapter Three
A Quick Look at Our History with Food

Food is everywhere. We can't go anywhere without seeing advertisements for food, or hearing someone talk about a favorite food or drink. Everywhere we look there are fast food restaurants. And, if you're like most women, you've tried a dozen different diets or certainly know someone who has.

Food is very much a part of who we are and our history. Long before gold coins came along, people traded food as a form of currency. Items like tea, sugar, and spices were exchanged for clothing, furniture, and animals.

In more modern times, the value of food has changed. Today, because it is so cheap and easy to get (at least, in the United States), we tend to think of food as something we deserve rather than something we need. The real problem in nutrition, however, is most people don't know how to eat. Funny as that sounds, it is sadly true. We super-size everything – eating and drinking too much, taking in too much junk food, and eating too little nutritious food. Most people who are unhealthy and/or overweight are so because they simply do not know how to choose healthy foods.

Being overweight (or significantly underweight) isn't the only health problem. A big mistake we make again and again is focusing on our appearance rather than how we feel. We're so worried about losing weight that, whether we're thin or heavy, we constantly diet and deny our bodies of proper nutrients. Junk food – as good as it might taste – is slowly destroying our bodies, health, and happiness.

1. Food on the Brain

Today, we have so many modern conveniences, such as refrigerators, ovens, and microwaves; it is almost impossible to imagine how early settlers once lived. There were no drive-thru restaurants or four-minute microwave meals. Cooking meals for the family was difficult work as preparation for meals began at 5:00 o'clock in the morning. Firewood had to cut and heavy iron kettles filled with water had to be hauled at great distances. Ovens were nothing more than holes in the wall. There were no temperatures gauges as we have on our ovens today, so young girls would stick their arm in the oven, above the flame, and count to 30. If they could not get to 30 before their skin was burning, they knew the oven was hot enough!

For early settlers, preparing food was an all-day chore. But once everyone was seated at the table, thanks and honor were given to those who made it all possible. No one ever ate out of boredom or while sitting in front of a television set. There were very few overweight settlers as eating was a privilege that came only after hard work. Although today – in the United States – we have the means to safely and easily cook, freeze, and store food; and although we have better, healthier, cleaner living conditions and healthier foods than ever before, we are actually becoming more overweight and unhealthy. Why?

We have food on the brain. If it seems we think too much about food, perhaps it is because images of food are everywhere. Did you know the average American child watches more than 10,000 food commercials each year? And that's just on television. But here is the really dangerous part. These are not commercials about eating fruits and vegetables. The commercials we are used to seeing show kids eating sugared cereals, fast foods, soft drinks, and candy in a fun and positive way. People are dancing with cartoons characters, and can win prizes if they eat or drink certain foods. Everyone in the commercials is having a great time. Just seeing the commercials makes us want to be part of that fun, doesn't it? Many commercials have misled kids to think that these foods are actually healthier than home-cooked meals.

We have never been more overweight and/or out of shape in the history of this country. Health experts have ranks child and adult obesity as the number one health problem in this country.

Simply put, when we consume more calories than we burn by exercising, we gain weight. The early settlers worked from sunrise to sunset, burning many, many calories. But today, because we have remote controls and cars and refrigerators, we don't have to (or want to) work nearly as hard as our ancestors did. And we are getting lazier and lazier. Just since the 1970s, we have become less active yet consume 200 calories more a day. As a result, we are gaining weight.

Though we have better medical care, cleaner living conditions, and more access to healthier foods than ever before, we're getting worse, not better. Here's why: We are eating too much, too fast. Only in the United States do restaurants have buffets (All You Can Eat!). We are offered super-sized deals (but who really loses?) where we almost feel guilty if we don't upgrade for an additional .40 cents.

Soft drinks used to be packaged in small eight-ounce bottles; today the most popular size is 34 ounces. According to the World Health Organization, Americans eat double and sometime triple the amount of food that people in other countries eat. But because it is so fast and relatively cheap to get food, and because our lifestyles are so busy, we all tend to eat too much. It may be fast and easy, but it is an unhealthy lifestyle that is carrying over into the lifestyles of our children.

We know this, yet it's so hard to walk away from yummy French fries.

Different things drive us to eat. We eat because we are bored, restless, sad, celebrating, nervous, or hungry. Food symbolizes many things to many people – food can mean family time, holiday parties, or comfort when we are lonely. Even certain colors can make you hungrier. In fact, studies have shown that the colors yellow, red, and orange trigger hunger with people. Now we know why most fast food restaurants are designed with those colors! The color green appeals to more healthful eaters, but beware! Sometimes this color can fool us into thinking that what we are eating is healthier than it really is. Colors, music, and packaging are

used in a way to make us feel hungry even when we are not. No surprise –
television is a huge hunger trigger.

Perhaps when you understand just how our food works for YOU it will enable
you to make better choices.

2. Understanding Fats, Protein, and Carbohydrates

To be a healthy, happy, successful, energized person, we need three things in
our diets: macronutrients, micronutrients and water. Because so many people do
not understand the real importance of food, we often chose diets that are not very
healthy. **Macronutrients** are carbohydrates, fat, and protein that help give us
energy, fight disease, build muscle, and rebuild body tissue. **Micronutrients** are
the vitamins and minerals we get from different foods to help keep our bodies
running like an efficient machine. The **nutrients** we get from food is absorbed by
the **organs** in our bodies, fueling us for the day. You've heard the expression, "you
are what you eat." This is definitely true!

We need to avoid fat because everything we have ever heard about fat is bad,
right? The truth is, fat is good for us. Everyone needs to have some fat in his or her
diet. The problem is Americans digest too much fat. When cooked, fat has a good
flavor and a smell most people like. Fat is what makes French fries nice and crispy
and helps make cookies chewy and gooey. That kind of fat, also known as
saturated fat, can be unhealthy for us if we eat too much of it. Have you ever
watched someone drain the grease from a skillet into a cup or jar after making
bacon? The fat takes on a solid form when kept at room temperature. Whereas
unsaturated fats (**monosaturated** and **polyunsaturated**) are in a liquid form as
olive oil, kanola oil, and peanut oil, to name a few.

What does fat do for us? Fat is our largest fuel tank, storing energy so we can
work and play all day long. It helps us focus at work, building brain cells and
helping to protect our skin against weather that is too hot or too cold. Fat acts as a
cushion for our organs, protecting our hearts, kidneys, and everything else in our
bodies from injury.

Of all the things we feed ourselves, carbohydrates may be the most
misunderstood. There are good **carbohydrates** and bad carbohydrates. Despite all
the negative things you have heard about carbohydrates, they are extremely
important for children and adults. They give us energy, help us think and keep our
bodies running healthily. But the wrong kind of carbohydrates can cause **insulin
surges** and unhealthy cravings. What does that mean?

Bad carbohydrates, like cakes and cookies, are mostly sugar. When we eat
these things, our bodies digest them very quickly and, then, believe that they need
more and more. Good carbohydrates, however, are **fiber**-filled so when it is eaten,
our bodies digest them slowly and evenly, leaving us feeling full and energized.
Fiber, such as apples, bran cereals, beans, and salads also provide our bodies with
added nutrients to fight unhealthy bacteria.

It is **proteins** that build muscles and fuel the development of organs in our bodies. Protein makes us strong and is very filling. Unlike sugary foods that allow us to eat and eat and eat, protein fills our stomachs and keeps us satisfied longer. Also unlike sugary-based foods, excess proteins in our bodies are not stored as fat. Instead, our bodies **excrete** it as waste. In other words, our bodies flush the extra protein out when we go to the bathroom.

It is estimated that pregnant women need 60 grams of protein during their pregnancy. But be careful. This isn't an absolute. Dependent upon you, your lifestyle, genetics, and medical history, you need to speak with your Team Baby about what is needed for a proper, balanced diet.

*Look to the list of healthy proteins for more options.

3. Vitamins and Minerals for a Stronger You

Consider this: from 1860 to 1865, the United States had a civil war. Northern states (the Union) and southern states (the Confederacy) fought with each other over slavery, the economy, and rights of each state. Many soldiers were killed and those who lived were often cold and hungry – very hungry because there wasn't enough food. In fact, the southern soldiers were **malnourished** (lacking proper vitamins and minerals) and were literally starving to death. The northern soldiers, however, were not malnourished.

Why were the Union soldiers healthier? Tomatoes! Yes, tomatoes helped the North win the Civil War.

What? Tomatoes helped win a war?

In many way, yes. The companies that canned tomatoes were in the northern states, and they sent their tomatoes to the Union Army. The tomatoes provided plenty of Vitamin C, among other nutrients, and gave the soldiers the strength to continue fighting. Because food is so plentiful for us today, it is hard to imagine being so exhausted and hungry. It is hard to imagine our bodies shutting down on us because we are malnourished. But there are actually stories of Confederate soldiers who surrendered to the Union side just so they could get something to eat.

Even though most Americans have enough to eat, some health experts argue that many of us are in very poor health and don't know it. Because we often eat junk food and neglect the important food groups such as fruits and vegetables, we can be lacking in proper nutrients. When our bodies do not get the proper amounts of vitamins and minerals, we are more likely to be sick, tired, lacking in energy, and inefficient in performing tasks (such as school work or chores).

So, what are **vitamins** and **minerals**?

Vitamins are **organic** substances, which means that they come from living things, such as fruits and vegetables. We need these vitamins to help prevent disease and have a normal growth rate and good **metabolism.** Vitamins are hard-working substances that can be divided into two groups based on the way they are absorbed into our bodies: They are fat-soluble or water-soluble. Vitamins A, D, E, and K are fat-soluble, which means that they are dissolved into the body's fat where they are stored. They come from meats, liver, egg yolks, oils, and some leafy green vegetables. Water-soluble vitamins, such as C and B, come from watery foods (oranges, tangerines, grapefruit) and are dissolved in water. This means each time we go to the bathroom, the vitamins are flushed through our systems. It is a reason why doctors urge us to take a lot of Vitamin C so we can replace the vitamin in our bodies. These vitamins help our immune systems fight diseases and infection.

Minerals come from non-living things, such as water and soil. But we can also get minerals from animals and plants as they absorb water, soil, and grass into their systems. The plants and animals pass these important nutrients on to us when we consume vegetables and/or meat. Again, there are two different kinds of minerals in our bodies. **Macrominerals** are composed of calcium, phosphorus, and magnesium. You have probably heard about calcium because it helps to build stronger bones and fight osteoporosis – a condition that affects bones as we get older, causing them to be brittle and break easily.

Microminerals (sodium, fluoride, potassium, chloride, iron, zinc, iodine, copper, manganese, chromium, selenium, molybdenum, arsenic, boron, nickel, and silicon) are all needed in the human body as well. Together, the macro- and microminerals create strong bones, teeth, and muscles and carry oxygen to cells through the blood.

Did you know that the color of a fruit or vegetable can be important to our diet? **Phytonutrients**, or phytos, are what give fruits and vegetables their colors. The general rule is, the darker the color, the better. For this reason, blueberries, pink grapefruit (not white), sweet potatoes and, yes, tomatoes, produce **antioxidants**, which removes junk from our bodies. Dark green veggies are best in the vegetable department. Spinach lettuce is much healthier for you than the light green iceberg lettuce.

How we feel, how we work, how we exercise and live all rely upon how well we feed ourselves.

4. You Are What You Drink

Liquid candy – that's what many health experts call carbonated sodas and sports drinks. We know soda drinks are unhealthy – they are bad for our skin, naturally dehydrate us and gives some people headaches – but many of us still drink "liquid candy." Additionally, there is an ingredient in soda called **phosphate**. It's phosphate that depletes the calcium in your bones, weakening them. And, of course, with the weakened bones comes the larger waistline – pre-pregnancy.

Because these drinks are tasty and easy to get, they are more popular than ever. A person who drinks a 20-ounce bottle of soda and/or sports drink a day is likely to gain a significant amount of weight but when that same person drinks water and/or milk instead, he/she tends to lose weight and feel better. One reason is that both milk and water make the drinker feel full, whereas the sugar in soda drinks will only make the thirsty person crave more and more.

If you are a caffeine drinker, you should know caffeine is an addictive drug that triggers a need within your body. Once you stop drinking it, you can get what is called "rebound" or "caffeine" headaches.

Many of the fruit drinks you see on the market today are not much better. Because the names of the drinks can be confusing, it is easy to think that the drinks are healthy. For example, Snapple and Minute Maid are very high in sugar. Many other drinks that call themselves fruit drinks have very little fruit in them: The main ingredient being sugar, not fruit. Sports drinks are popular because kids (and their parents) think it must be healthy if it is called a sports drink. However, both Powerade and Gatorade are high in **glucose, fructose**, and **high-fructose corn syrup**. In other words: sugar and chemicals. Nothing beats milk, water, or 100 percent fruit juice.

Question:
"I've just become pregnant and like to drink herbal teas. Are there any teas that are dangerous to the baby or that I should avoid?"

Answer:
Because the safety and effectiveness of herbal supplements really have not been studied in pregnancies, it is always necessary to be cautious. You need to speak to your OB/GYN first and foremost. But the March of Dimes, United Way and scores of other health agencies urge mothers-to-be to read the labels and avoid herbal supplements such as:

Arnica	Foxglove	Nutmeg	Tansy ragwort
Black Cherry	Gordolobo	Oleander	Tonka bean
Bloodroot	Groundsel	Pennyroyal	T'u-san-chi
Buckthorn	Jimsonweed	Periwinkle	Water Hemlock
Burdock root	Lobelia	Poke root	Woodruff
Blue Cohosh	Mandrake	Sassafras	Wormwood
Comfrey	Melilot	Senna	Yohimbe
Elderberry	Mormon tea	Snakeroot	

This is just a sampling. For more information, check out the website: www.worldhostone.com to learn more about what you are drinking.

*Consuming more than three cups of coffee a day has been linked with infertility! A woman who is already pregnant may deliver an underweight baby and in more extreme cases, where women consumed 8 to 25 cups of coffee a day, there was a higher instance of babies born with birth defects.

*A study with Harvard University's Nurses' Health Study found that women who drank four or more cans of soda a day were 16 to 44 percent more likely to develop high blood pressure. The cause? Surprisingly, not the caffeine but the sodium – a well-known blood pressure booster. Researchers also believe that corn syrup may be a contributing factor. …Just another reason to lay off the junk and drink more water!

5. Diets, Diets, Everywhere Diets!

Don't believe the hype: Food is not our enemy. As much as we love food, we hate it. We blame food for our weaknesses or being overweight. We use food to reward ourselves for something and later punish ourselves for eating it. Most American adults have tried at least one diet in hopes of losing weight quickly. Health experts remind us again and again that weight loss should be a slow, gradual process. After all, we don't put on those extra pounds overnight. Still, we try to lose weight quickly. Let's take a look at some of those "quick fix" diets and talk about why they don't work in the long run.

High Protein/Low Carbohydrates

You may have heard about diets that say you can eat all the meat and protein products (like cheese) you want but you must not eat very many carbohydrates (such as bread, pasta, and cereal). These diets claim that Americans are so fat because we eat too many carbohydrates that raises blood sugar and causes our bodies to produce too much insulin. Insulin is the hormone that produces glucose for our cells. This is why we gain weight.

The high protein/low carbohydrate diets claim that fewer carbohydrates mean less insulin so our bodies use (and burn) body fat instead and we lose weight. But the truth is, most of the weight loss is water weight. Even worse, this diet causes some muscle loss – we want to lose fat, not muscle.

This diet also limits the amount of vegetables and fruits which means we are missing important nutrients. While we can lose weight quickly on this plan, the weight loss is only temporary.

High Fiber/Low Fat

This diet claims that fiber is very filling and it takes longer to chew which means we probably consume less calories. When we feel full, we are likely to consume fewer calories, which means we can lose weight. Lots of fruits and vegetables are required for this diet which does provide plenty of vitamins and minerals, but there is such a thing as too much of a good thing.

By eating more fiber and less fat and protein, we can probably lose some weight but the risks are diarrhea, gas, bloating, and nausea. Too much fiber can be very difficult for the human body to handle for a long period of time. And, like most diets, any weight loss is only temporary.

Fruit Smoothies/Meal Supplements

You may have seen the commercials for diets that promise weight loss if we have two smoothies-like drinks with fruity or chocolate flavors a day with a reasonably-sized meal for dinner. Like any diet that limits entire food groups, this diet is low in calories. It is likely that we will be very hungry. If we feel starved, our metabolism slows down, making weight loss even harder. This is a good example of our minds and bodies working together.

That's right. Our brains send messages to our bodies all the time. If we don't eat enough, our brains send messages that it is starving. Instantly, our bodies go into high alert – protecting the fat it already has by slowing down metabolism to stop fat loss. Our bodies and brains do not know we have refrigerators full of food. They only know we are starving our bodies and they fight to save the fat. That's why starvation or food depravation is never a good diet plan.

Herbal Appetite Suppressants or Stimulants

Many people believe if they are taking herbs – natural ingredients – to lose weight, it is safe. Not all herbs, however, are safe. The Food and Drug Administration (FDA) was established by Congress in 1929 to watch over and regulate all drug products sold to the American public. But because herbs are not considered drugs or medicine, the FDA did not have control of their sale as diet aids. Then, several people died from the herb called ephedra. Ephedra, among many herbs that promises to burn fat and suppress appetite, has been responsible for more than 16,000 people having heart attacks, seizures, strokes and other ailments. More than 200 people have died. Because the herb causes your heart to beat faster and stimulates the nervous system, people may experience tremors, dizziness, nervousness, and chest pain. There is an easier and much safer way to lose weight!

Question:
"I was taking Hydroxycut when I found out I'm pregnant. Did I do any damage?"

Answer:
First, you need to make an appointment and speak with your OB/GYN. But, until that time, I would not worry about this as you have (I hope) stopped taking the supplement. That said, permit me to go on a health tangent. The dangers of taking 'fat burning' and 'energy boosting' supplements are far reaching. There are record numbers of people who have suffered strokes, heart attacks, irreversible heart valve damage, and death.

No matter your situation, desire to lose weight, or reach a final goal, there is no excuse for taking these dangerous supplements. And we are in a dire situation in this nation as so many Americans simply do not understand basic nutritional facts and believe that if a product is on the market it must be safe. With new products like Monster, Red Bull, and now Cocaine on the market, our children are in terrible danger.

Don't worry about what you have done. Now focus on living a healthy lifestyle and promise that, for the sake of your baby, you will not return to these products once the baby is born.

The best diet? The early settlers had that figured out. They worked hard and ate well-balanced meals each day. Today, health experts tell us to eat five to six small meals a day. As we know, the ideal way to live a healthy lifestyle is to eat a healthy, *balanced* diet and exercise! When we sit up, roll over, climb stairs, mop the floor, rake the leaves, even fold laundry that requires muscles. The more we exercise our muscles, the stronger we get. Even better, the more we exercise our muscles, the more we will burn fat. Yes, even while we sleep. Because muscle burns fat naturally, we can be sure our exercise routines and balanced diets will help us lose weight and keep it off. No chancey diets, just natural weight control and good health.

So, why am I sharing this information with pregnant readers? Certainly not to diet! But the best way to make you understand the importance of eating balanced diets and keep you away from the notion of 'dieting' is to let you read and understand how unbalanced the gimmicky diets actually are. The more you read about early settlers, the more you realize how misguided our eating habits (and lifestyle) are today. Now that you are in your most maternal, "earthy" state, this is the time to get back to the basics!

6. Sugar, Sugar, Everywhere Sugar

Humans have always enjoyed sweets. Natural sugars, such as honey, have been part of our diets since prehistoric times. **Sucrose**, which is a refined sugar, was first refined from sugarcane, a giant sweet grass found in warm climate. Today, Hawaii is one of the largest growers of sugarcane. In the 18th Century (that's over 300 years ago), farmers discovered sugar could also be **extracted** from sugar beets – a root plant that grows in the ground. **Fructose**, extracted from fruit and honey, and **corn syrup**, which comes from cornstarch, are two more natural sweeteners. In fact, if you read the ingredients on most cereal boxes, cookie packages and bread labels, you will find corn syrup as one of the main ingredients because it is inexpensive to make.

While sugar is a carbohydrate that offers energy, the calories are empty calories. That means, the sugar is instantly **dispersed** into your blood system and stored as fat. It offers no nutritional value, which means you do not get any needed vitamins or minerals from sugar. Too many sugary drinks, cakes, and candy do nothing but add fat and calories to your diet, not to mention what sugar does to your teeth.

Many people turn to **artificial** sweeteners as a way to avoid extra, unwanted calories. You may have heard of saccharin or aspartame. **Saccharin**, also known as Sweet 'n Low, is made with chemicals and has been found to cause cancer in laboratory rats. While there are no known cases of a human getting cancer as a result of using saccharin, health experts stress that natural foods are always best. **Aspartame**, also known as Equal or Nutrasweet, is very popular but has possible health risks as well. People who suffer from severe allergies, migraine headaches, or other head pain are advised to avoid these products since they tend to trigger greater head pain.

Because there are now so many kinds of sugars or sweeteners, it can be confusing to choose the right ones. For example, corn syrup is a naturally occurring sweet but high-fructose corn syrup is chemically processed and potentially very upsetting to your body. Because your body is unable to break down this chemical properly, the fat level in your blood is raised. A sure sign your body is getting too much **high-fructose corn syrup** in your waist (pre-pregnancy!). Your middle is a favorite place for your body to store fat and health experts are noticing that adults as well as children and teenagers are getting thicker (keeping more fat) in the middle sections than at any other time in history. While this is not the time in your life to be worrying about extra fat on your mid-section, this is the time to be thinking about healthful foods and drinks. Loading up on empty calories does not benefit you or the baby.

It may be harder than you think to eat less sugar because sugar is addictive. That's right! There is a chemical in our brains that tells us we want more and more sugar, and the more you eat it, the more you want it. By learning to eat natural, sweet **alternatives**, you can lose weight, have better nutrition, and train your brain to choose healthier foods. So, is sugar bad for you? No, but like most things, natural foods in moderation are best. To say that another way: eating reasonable amounts of natural foods, including sugar, is always healthier.

Some alternatives:
Try slicing up some apples. Sprinkle cinnamon on top. Freeze fruit juice on a hot day and eat it like a popsicle. Try yogurt with fruit or squirt lemon into plain water to give it more flavor. Sprinkle cocoa mix on a banana or freeze grapes. There are all kinds of healthy sweeteners that are natural and delicious. Go for it!

7. Learning How to Eat: Tricks of the Meal
Most families today have very little time to sit down at the table and eat as a family. This is the reason fast food restaurants are so successful and it also why so many people have poor eating habits. We eat on the go, cramming food in our mouths, and gobbling everything up as quickly as possible. We don't care if it's even good for us, we just want and need to eat quickly.

The result? We are overweight, unhealthy, and (no surprise) have very poor table manners. Here are some tips to help you eat better, be healthier, and enjoy your food (and the companionship of family and friends) much more:

Portion Size

The biggest problem we have today is the amount of food we eat. Make a fist with your hand and look at it. That is the size of meat needed for a meal, nothing bigger. Now, cup your hands together. Your portion of vegetables should fit neatly into your (two) cupped hands. And for carbohydrates like pasta, rice, or potatoes? The size of just one cupped hand is needed for carbohydrates. That is a well-balanced, well-proportioned meal. The same rules for portion size apply to adults and children. And, remember, just because you're pregnant doesn't mean you get to make two fists. Just one.

*Pregnant women are often told that red meat is an excellent source of protein – it is – but rather than using moderation, gorge themselves on an all-meat diet. Here's what you need to know.

Slow Down

Rush, rush, rush. Everyone is in a rush but you should always take time to slow down and sit down while you eat. Do not stand at the kitchen counter. Studies have shown people tend to eat much faster and much more when standing. Let your digestive system do its work while you sit and enjoy a meal slowly. Here are some fun "slow down" things to try at the dinner table. While the ideas may seem silly, you are almost forced to slow down. If you already have kids, they will LOVE this new game!

- Try using chopsticks to handle your food.
- Let one minute pass before each new bite.
- Hold your fork in the opposite hand with which you usually eat.
- Put down your fork each time you have taken a bite and do not pick it up again until you have chewed and swallowed the bite.

Smaller Bites

Each meal should last at least 20 minutes. If you are with friends/ family, the meal should last 40 minutes. This way you know you are eating slowly, engaging in conversation – that is, talking and listening and not just shoveling food in your mouth – and truly enjoying the food. Try cutting your food into little pieces. Remember, the bigger the bites, the harder it is for your body to break up and digest the food.

Chew More

With each bite you take, whether you are eating an apple slice or a piece of bread, try to count as you chew. Count from ten to 20 chews with each bite. And be sure to swallow that bite before putting another into your mouth. You will be amazed how hard it is at first to chew so much and you will also see how quickly you've been eating.

Look at the Clock

Are you really hungry? Or, are you just eating because of something you saw on television? Are you bored? Restless? Listen to your body and determine if you really are hungry. Look at the clock to see what time it is. If it is late in the afternoon, make yourself a light snack so you won't spoil your dinner. Or just have a glass of water. It will satisfy your urge to eat or drink something and it will be good for you.

8. Foods to Be Avoided

In January 2006, I traveled to the EPA (Environmental Protection Agency) headquarters in Raleigh, N.C. to testify before a subcommittee on the dangerous levels of mercury and other hazardous materials emitted into our air, water, and soil. Whatever it was I thought I knew before going to the hearing, I was horrified as I sat listening to experts from around the nation testify on the levels of reported mercury in our fishing waters.

Two years prior, in March 2004, the FDA and EPA issued joint guidelines regarding eating fish during pregnancy. Women who are pregnant, nursing, or merely thinking about having children are urged to eat no more than two servings of fish each week in order to protect developing babies from high levels of potentially brain-damaging mercury. What I learned in 2006 made me question the guidelines as they stand today. We are allowing dangerous levels on toxins into our environment, allowing breaks for industries/factories in the name of business. But who pays for this in the long run? While there are most definitely benefits from eating seafood, you must heavily consider the risk of eating contaminated fish or shellfish. It's another great reason to consider organic!

Stay away from shark, swordfish, king mackerel, or golden or white snapper (tilefish) because they contain high levels of mercury. The most popular fish is albacore or white tuna but this has reportedly more mercury than canned tuna. It is not recommended that you consume more than 6 ounces per week. Tuna steak also has higher levels of mercury than canned tuna.

While shrimp, canned light tuna, salmon, pollock, fish sticks and catfish have the lower levels of mercury, please be cautious of what you chose and how much you eat.

You may also want to rethink your choice in cheese and dairy products. According to the U.S. Department of Agriculture, listereriosis, a food-borne illness with flu- or cold-like symptoms that might otherwise be written off as nothing more, can cause premature labor, miscarriage, and severe illness to the baby.

Pasteurized milk kills the listeria organism but unpasteurized soft cheeses and other unpasteurized dairy products, can harbor it, causing terrible problems. Cheeses such as Brie, Camembert, feta, goat, Montrachet, Neufchatel, and queso fresco should be avoided as well as the semi-soft cheeses Asiago, blue, brick, Gorgonzola, Havarti, Muenster, and Roquefort.

9. Healthy Choices

Take some time to review the things you have learned about carbohydrates, proteins, sugars, and fat. Take an honest look how many sugary drinks you consume. We all get very busy with housework, work, our children, and grocery shopping. It is all too easy to get into the habit of buying food that other family members will eat rather than foods we *should* eat. But now is the time to make life changes that will help and inspire and energize everyone.

Take a look at the food pyramid or log on to www.choosemyplate.gov.

Trust me when I say, children also want to make lifestyle changes. They may resist the food change in the beginning but they really do want to eat more healthily.

From time to time, I receive questions from children who want to make those lifestyle changes which I love because it is a reminder to us all how brilliant children are.

Question:

Yes, but my little sister is a picky eater and doesn't like anything! What can we do?

Ask your parent or guardian to sit down with you and your brothers and sisters and pick out meals from the cookbook. If you don't have any picture cookbooks, maybe you can borrow some at the library. Pick out meals that look good to you, are well-balanced, and that everyone likes. Now, make your grocery list and get started.

How do I know what is a good carbohydrate and a bad one?

Brownies, cakes, and cookies that are loaded with fats and sugar are not the best carbohydrates. They offer little nutritional value, as do french fries and potato chips that are dripping in grease and fat. Take a look at the carbohydrates list below to find solid, healthy foods that will give you energy and power.

Carbohydrates – Ultimate Energy Foods – easily converted

Breads –
   Bagel, mini, whole-grain (½ bagel 1 ounce)

Starchy Vegetables (½ cup)
   Corn

Bread, whole-grain (1 slice – 1 ounce)
Muffin, high fiber (½ small)
Pita, whole-grain, 6-inch (½ pita = 1 ounce) cup)
Tortilla, whole grain, 6–inch (1)

Peas, green
Potato, baked (3 ounce)
Potato, sweet, mashed (1/3
Squash, winter (1 cup)

Cereal –
Cereal, cooked (½ cup)
Cereal, dry, unsweetened (½ cup)
Cereal, granola (¼ cup)

Fruit --
Apple
Applesauce (½ cup)
Apricot halves, dried (7)
Banana (½ large)
Blueberries or blackberries

Legumes – (1/3 cup)

Beans, black
Beans, kidney
Beans, lima
Beans, pinto
Beans, white
Lentils
Peas, black-eyed
melon
Peas, split

(3/4 cup)
Cantaloupe (1/3 melon or
    1 cup of cubes)
Cherries (12)
Grapefruit (½ cup)
Grapes (½ cup)
Honeydew melon (1/8 of

or 1 cup of cubes)
Kiwi (1)
Mango (½)
Orange (medium)

Whole Grains (½ cup)
Pasta, whole-wheat, cooked
Bulgar, cooked

Crackers and Snack Foods
Crackers (6)
Melba toast (5)
Popcorn, air-popped (3 cups)
Pretzels (¾ ounce)
Rye crisp or Wasa-type crackers (2 to 4)
Tortilla chips (8)

Rice (1/3 cup)
Brown, rice
White, rice

Is meat protein?
Protein, like carbohydrates, is very important for building muscles and tissues, and it comes it a variety of foods.   Yes, meat is a very popular source of protein but you will be surprised by the other kinds of foods with protein you and your family can eat.

Proteins

Dairy
Cottage cheese, nonfat (½ cup)
Milk, 1% (8 oz)
Yogurt, plain nonfat (1 cup)

Meat
Beef, lean (4 oz)
Egg white (1)
Egg, whole (1)
Fish, tuna (4 oz)
Poultry, breast, no skin
(4 oz)
Salmon (4 oz)

Whole Grains
Whole-wheat bread (1 slice)
Pasta (I cup)

Cereals
Cereal, grain, (1 cup) with ½ cup of milk

Legumes
kidney beans (½ cups)
Tofu, firm (3 oz)

*Also, peanut butter (2 tbsp.) and nuts or sunflower seeds (1 oz) are excellent protein sources!

I like to eat cookies and muffins. If I want to eat healthy does that mean I can't eat them because of fat?

There are good fats and bad fats. You need to stay away from greasy fast foods and things cooked with butters and lard. Nuts, egg yolk, tuna, avocado and seeds are considered to be smart fats. For cooking, you can use olive oil and canola oil in replace of margarine and Crisco. When you sit down to talk about cooking meals, be sure to show these lists to your adult to help in making wiser, healthier choices.

My teacher says we should learn how to cut unnecessary fat from our diets. How can we do that and still have good fat?

Instead of drinking whole milk, switch to low-fat milk. Exchange whole-milk yogurts and high-fat cheeses for low-fat. Instead of eating french fries, try sweet potatoes and use low-fat yogurt instead of sour cream on your baked potato. Use olive oil on pasta or breads instead of butter and try hummus instead of salad dressing.

Be sure to limit your intake of beef, try turkey instead of chicken, and always try to have white-meat poultry rather than the dark meat. Try a veggie burger or tofu instead of hamburger. Many kids are unwilling to try new things simply because it looks different but it can be fun to try new things with other people. With your family, find pictures of foods that look good and make the meal together.

When you know exactly what is in the meal and how it was prepared – especially if you helped -- you may like it all the more.

How do I know if something is healthy?

The best way to learn more about the foods you and your family eat is to read the labels on the food. As you have already learned, you want to stay away from foods that list sugar as one of the main ingredients, particularly if it is high-fructose corn syrup. Remember that you want your food to be as **organic** as possible. In other words, foods that are not made by people: carrots, apples, oranges, nuts, raisins, fish and meats, whole-grain cereals. Did you ever read the ingredient label on an orange? There isn't one! Because it isn't made from anything except sunshine, water, and orange.

I want to eat organic but it just doesn't take good!

This is a myth swallowed whole by junk food eaters. The truth is, without the use of fertilizers to speed the growth of vegetables or preservatives to make the shelf life of the product longer, the true flavor of the food is compromised. The more chemicals are used to enhance the food, the less healthy and tasty it actually is.

*See Chapter 11: I Want the Change My Eating Habits to learn how to break the fast food habit.

10 Rules for the Table

1. Only healthy drinks will be served. No sugary drinks allowed!
2. Limit the amount of salt used. Experiment with other seasonings for meats and vegetables.
3. Think like a rabbit! Try to begin your meals with a small salad. By eating a small salad before the main meal is served, you will get much needed minerals and vitamins. You will be less likely to fill up on the heavier foods.
4. Talk about the meal, making sure everyone knows the nutritional benefits of what you are eating and what all the food groups are. This is a fun way for you, little brother and sisters, and even your parents/guardians to learn more about the food groups. Quiz them on what macro- and micronutrients are.
5. No negative conversations at the dinner table. This means no tattling, no arguing, and no complaining!
6. Set a timer for 30 to 40 minutes. This is the time your family should have together at the table. Even if you need to bring notes to the table for things to talk about, be sure the family sits together until the timer bell rings. Soon enough, your family will want to sit together longer than the timer says.

7. Practice eating slowly together. For fun, have everyone use his or her fork with the opposite hand he or she usually uses and make everyone count how many times he or she chews.

8. Take turns talking about how your day was. When it is someone else's turn to talk, use this time to be a good listener and ask questions. You will be amazed what you learn about your family during this time.

9. Discuss what the next meal should be, letting everyone have a vote. Be careful! Don't let your little sister ruin your good efforts by ordering a pizza. Be sure the adults control the vote by ensuring that vegetables, protein, and carbohydrates are presented.

10. Talk about one thing outside your family – a news story about another person or
place. Perhaps you and your family members could take turns telling about something in the newspaper or on TV or that you learned at school or work. Older family members can help younger ones so everyone has a turn. Good food and good conversation go together.

Chapter Four
What Your Trainer Isn't Telling You

If you're already working out, you're most likely reading this book because you want to know what exercises are safe and what are not. You want to know about heart rate, inner core temperature, muscle recovery and muscle memory. (Hang on, you'll get all the information you need!). But if you've been sedentary most or all of your life, you want and need to know how to get started. On that note: Hurray! Good for you!

Whatever your physical state, everyone will be quick to applaud your efforts for getting or staying in shape while pregnant. Trainers, doctors, training buddies, friends, and family will all offer advice, even commiserate with you as to how hard it is to find motivation while pregnant. Okay, here's the real deal: Now is the time to get into the exercise routine because this really is the easiest time of your baby time. Your baby is snuggly safe inside of you. Finding time and motivation from being sleep deprived or feeling out of shape will be your greatest challenges after the baby is born.

Thanks to the highly profiled confessions of celebrity moms, such as Brooke Shields, women are finally talking about the fact that's it's not all daisies and lollipops once baby is born. With that realization (for some) comes a lot of guilt. Somehow, they feel they have failed Motherhood 101 by feeling blue, depressed, and ugly.

Question:
"I want to work out but I just can't find the motivation. I am 14 weeks pregnant and I'm just so tired all the time."

Answer:
"You better get motivated now, Momma, or you're REALLY going to be tired once the baby comes!"

That was just the first sentence to a very long "What to do to get motivated" answer. I've broken that particular answer into the following sections. But the real point here is if you've decided you'll get in shape *after* the baby is born, that you'll worry about your fitness level *after* the baby is born, that you'll get more energy *after* the baby is born, you're in for a very rude and difficult awakening.

As you've read, I did train throughout my second and third pregnancies and do honestly believe I had more energy than the average mom. But, briefly, I had deluded myself into thinking I had everything under control after my second child was born. I was juggling my training, writing career, bobsledding, travel, marriage, and my one daughter. It wasn't always pretty but I was hanging in there. Then, baby number two came along.

I still remember one particular trip I had to make to New York. My husband was putting in long hours at work so I decided that I would drive, taking my babies with me so that we could have quality time. I also -- for reasons I now do not understand – decided to take Nala, our beloved Shepherd mix.

Actually, the trip was okay. Coming back was a nightmare. In desperation, I'd broken my cardinal rule of no fast-food with my babies and bought some disgusting kid meal. My thinking was it would break up the present mood and give them something to focus on other than screaming.

A chicken nugget food fight broke out – the little rats knew Mommy couldn't get to them while driving – and Nala, queasy from car motion and nugget aroma wafting through the car, puked on the floor of the front seat. I yelled and the girls started crying. That with puppy barf and fried grease filling my nostrils was just about all I could take. I started crying. I found myself pressing forward, so absolutely eager to be able to work with my trainer – in silence – focusing on something physically demanding and challenging to work out my stress and frustrations rather than focusing on the emotionally demanding things – like soaring chicken nuggets and puppy puke.

You will read countless books and magazine articles that will tell you that in order to find the motivation to work out, you should focus on an event, such as an upcoming wedding or bathing suit season. You should tape a picture to your refrigerator of your pre-pregnant figure or of a model/actress you admire. The reality is, that's not going to help you. After a while, you'll ignore the picture on the refrigerator and you'll begin justifying how to get out of or get around the whole special event issue. In addition, it will make you focus on a non-pregnant form which does no one any good. You need to focus on working out because you need to, because it will make you happier, healthier, and stronger for your baby. That said, your biggest problem is finding the motivation and energy to work out. Listed below are some training tips and healthful advice that will reduce your stress (about working out), re-energize you, and arm your body with what you need to have better workouts.

1. What to Do

In the second half of this book, particular exercise and how to perform them will be laid out. But the real key is finding what you like. Far too many women mindlessly exercise because that's what everyone else is doing. But if you don't like aerobics, or cycling, or running, or kickboxing, where's your motivation?

You can go to the gym everyday but if you can't stand your workouts, you will never really succeed.

Trainers are conditioned to teach you how to perform specific functions and work various muscle groups. The good trainers will explain to you the benefits of these actions while you are exercising. But too few ask you, "So, what do you like to do?" and "What are your physical goals?"

I am always happily surprised to learn how many women wish they could run a 5k race or a half-marathon but are too embarrassed to tell anyone. For them, it seems like a ridiculous dream.

One woman once said, "The only way I would ever run (jog) is if someone was chasing me. I do NOT run." Today, she is training for a half-marathon!

1. But I'm pregnant! I can't do anything, right? Wrong. Tell your trainer or training buddy your fitness dream. You will never succeed in your workouts if you do not like what you are doing. You can simulate "in training" workouts while pregnant.
2. Make the goals realistic. You're pregnant. The idea here is to give you something fun to think about while training. Obviously, ice skating or downhill skiing is out!
3. Set a realistic timetable. While pregnant, you are simply gearing up for that sport or race you've been thinking about. Now, you can slowly and carefully begin to work muscles and get into a routine so that when baby is born, you will be ready to get serious!

2. Water: It's Highly Underrated!

The number one thing both trainers and nutritionists tell their clients is, "Be sure to drink plenty of water." They say it once and don't really approach the subject again. We all nod in agreement. Yes, yes, water is good … and go about our day.

So, why is water so great? When you drink water, it cleans the waste and unneeded toxins out of your body. It helps your body digest and move food more easily through your intestines and other body organs. It helps reduce constipation and bloat – two biggies while pregnant. Once you've begun a water-drinking habit, this will help you after the baby is born as well. When you breastfeed, your body will want to store fat. Drinking water is the best and most natural way to rid yourself of excess waste and toxins.

Just as fats, carbohydrates, and protein fuel your body, water makes your skin smooth, helps your muscles and joints move, keeps you energized and alert. It also keeps you from overeating. When you drink plenty of water, you feel full and are less likely to snack.

Water will help with morning sickness. Many women report craving salts (sodium) as a way to ease an upset stomach but it is the salt/sodium that triggers higher instances of morning sickness.

Does it seem like you get cramps a lot when you are running? This can mean you are not properly hydrated. Your muscles will begin to cramp when they want and need more water. Got a stitch in your side? It may mean you need more water in your diet. Believe it or not, the majority of Americans are dehydrated – meaning their bodies want and need more water. Both muscles and the brain are made up of 70 to 75 percent water. Our bodies need and crave water.

Are you constantly licking your lips and requiring lip moisturizers? Do your hands feel particularly dry? These are also classic symptoms of being naturally dehydrated.

So, how do you know when you are or aren't getting enough? Again, check the urine. Your kidneys act as a filter, draining water and waste products, safely keeping your blood cells and the larger protein molecules circulating throughout your body, and storing it in your bladder. But your body can only work with what you give it. If your body is naturally dehydrated, most of the water you do have will be absorbed back into the blood, making your kidneys work overtime and leaving your urine far more concentrated with by-products than it's supposed to be. Eventually, organs will shut down if not given water.

*It is important to note that other factors, such as diet, kidney function, and medications may affect the color/odor of your urine. If you are drinking enough water and notice dark yellow to reddish colored urine, you need to see your doctor.

3. What and When to Eat

Okay, here's the setup. You walk into your local gym and a very cute, 20-year-old fitness trainer with 8% body fat enthusiastically greets you at the door. "Hi, I'm Perky Sue, here to pump and pep you up!!"

Ugh.

Perky Sue may be pumped and pepped because she's 20, has no junk in her truck, isn't pregnant, and can exist on Red Bull and Ding Dongs. The rest of us human beings– particularly women – have other issues. One being anemia (see #4).

Now that you are pregnant, you need to focus on your diet. Again, writing in a journal is a great way to monitor just how much junk you actually take in. After one week, find a nutritionist in your area, set up an appointment and together, the two of you can take a hard look at your eating habits. You will be amazed by how much better you feel, sleep, exercise, and even communicate with other people when you are well nourished.

You may be resistant to the idea – perhaps you are embarrassed, short on time or money – but you will be doing yourself and the baby a great service by speaking with a professional and I don't think Perky Sue is the one for you.

To remind you:

The American Dietetic Association requires a four-year degree and a 9 to 12 month internship to qualify for the registered dietician (RD) credential, and candidates must pass a credited examination. Many RDs work in hospitals or other health-care facilities. To find a credited RD, log on to www.eatright.org.

A certified nutritionist must have a science or education in nutrition and take/pass an examination with the American Associations of Clinical Nutritionists (IAACN) to become an official CCN – certified clinical nutritionist. CCNs analyze how food affects you/your body and tailor a more suitable diet for your health and medical needs. To find a CCN near you, call (972) 407-9089

4. Inner Core Temperature

Ahh! My most favorite and popular topic in regards to exercise and pregnancy. Pay attention because this may be the very best advice you ever receive and it's certainly one that very, very few trainers and coaches talk to their clients/athletes about.

Unfortunately, most medical professionals and fitness experts tend to give the standard answer when it comes to pregnant athletes and spend very little time learning how to safely train a mom-to-be!

So what is your inner core temperature? Before I answer that, let me share with you my first experience with the rectal thermometer. I was at the MetroHealth Hospital, in the research laboratory when it was first presented to me.

"You want me to put that where?!?!?!"

There are certain things that neither God nor my Momma intended to be done to me, and sticking a long, reed-thin object attached to a temperature gauge on wheels up my behind was tops on the list. I eyed the research assistant skeptically.

You can just forget that, sister. I wouldn't even stick that in my ear.

At that point, I'd been hooked up to fetal and heart monitors, EKG leads, and oxygen masks in order to read how my body was reacting to specific workouts. We had wanted and needed to know how my body responded but more importantly how Katie, my bobsled baby, was doing.   It was explained to me that there was really no better way of monitoring her comfort level than getting a proper read on my inner core temperature.

My what!? Mind you, I was still staring at the long, skinny thing they wanted me to put in my rear end. I'd had my body fat analyzed with the underwater testing, been poked, prodded, had blood withdrawn and was constantly being weighed and measured, and I really didn't mind. But this ….?

Babies have no way to sweat, thus no natural way to cool or regulate their own body temperature. At all stages of pregnancy, the baby's temperature is one degree Celcius higher than the mother's. Avoiding fetal heat stress is very important during the first trimesters because that is the critical period in the development of the spinal cord. It is also another reason why so many physicians are concerned about when a pregnant mother gets a high fever.

Fetal disorders of the central nervous system have been connected to high maternal temperature from illness or warm water exposure. If you overheat, your baby has no mechanism for getting rid of excessive heat (like perspiration), and so relies solely on the mother to monitor temperature.

"Can't I just tell how hot I am by how much I'm sweating?"

"How do I take my inner core temperature? Can't I just use the kind you stick in your ear?"

No and no.

You will need to buy a rectal thermometer and pack it in your gym bag. Whether you are running bleachers, working out at the gym or dojo, hiking in the woods, cycling, or walking around the neighborhood, you will check your inner core temperature by way of rectal measurement every 20-30 minutes, dependent upon your level of exertion.

You do not want your inner core temperature to go beyond 101 degree F!

I've known women who hid behind bushes, ran into public bathrooms, crouched behind cars and ran out of busy aerobic classrooms to check their inner core temperature in the locker room. I don't care about the wheres, but I do want to impress upon you the importance of the whys.

You simply cannot feel your own forehead to determine just how hot you've become. As we've previously discussed, your inner core temperature will spike throughout your workout.

If you are hovering around 101 degree F during your workout, you need to back off. Get a drink of water and bring down the cardio level. Allow yourself to rest, cool down (internally) before you begin again.

In my kickbox classes, my students always tease me about how mean I am. I don't let people cheat themselves and firmly believe that if you've come to work – we should be working. But when it comes to pregnant women and inner core temperature, I am very watchful. There is no need to "push through" a specific exercise if you're working too hard or breathing harder than normal.

DO NOT get into a competition with other people.

Like Olympian Michelle Rohl, I have my own bad experience. I had been training on the VersaClimber, having already finished sprint sets on the bicycle and lunges with weights. I was dangerously hot but I had not stopped to check my inner core temperature. It was the one AND ONLY stupid mistake I made during my training while pregnant with Katie. Dr. Clapp and his assistant, Dr. Kathleen Little, had been monitoring my progress. I was strong and admittedly, was showing off. I had a false sense of security by their presence, believing that nothing bad could happen while they observed me. While they waited for me to give the sign of "peaking" I carried on. Dr. Little suddenly asked me to step down and had me sit while she pulled Dr. Clapp to the side. Sitting there, I suddenly realized how hot I had become, how hard I had been working, and then I realized they were having me sit there for a reason.

Katie's heart rate had slowed suddenly while my heart rate soared. I had held my heart rate at a high level for too long. The minutes dragged on miserably until they told me everything was normal again. I was so miserable and disappointed by my own poor lack of judgment, I did not work out for a few days after that, terrified that I had harmed Katie.

Learn from this story. Buy yourself a rectal thermometer and be diligent about checking your own temperature. Record the times and temperature along with what your activities were.

Remember that you are exercising for the health of both you and the baby. If you have to sit down, cool off, or walk out of a class – who cares? Safety is your number one issue here.

Use good judgment. Exercising mothers-to-be tend to be good about monitoring themselves. In studies, pregnant exercisers who chose their own exercise pace, as well as women who were held to a constant pace throughout gestation, were more likely to keep their body temperature well within safe limits.

5. Heart Rate

Every time I went to Clapp's research facility, I would turn in my exercise and diet log books. With the information I had gathered from the research program, I felt more comfortable training on my own. Whether I ran or biked, after a warm-up period, I would watch my heart rate. While most of the women I've talked to had been told to keep their heart rates under 140 bpm, my heart rate was typically higher. I was more concerned with my core temperature.

Question:
"My doctor told me to stop exercising when my heart started to really pound. But I get out of breath so fast that anytime I do anything, it seems like my heart is pounding. What can I do?"

Answer:
This is a common complaint. Now that you are pregnant, you blood and oxygen flow are different, thus, you will often find yourself out of breath just walking to the mailbox. Fear not. This is only temporary. And in no way does this mean you have to stop exercising. Let's talk about working out in the safety zone for recreational and elite athletes.

With new ACOG (American College of Obstetricians and Gynecologists) guidelines, more doctors are educating themselves about exercise and pregnancy, the point of exhaustion or breathlessness. In the past, medical and safety issues regarding pregnant exercisers have been focused on high body temperature, reduced delivery of oxygen and nutrients to the baby, stress to the body, and the effects of higher heart rates on the baby.

When talking to elite athletes, doctors tend to give the, "you know your own body, use discretion" advice. But what of recreational athletes or the sedentary-turned-exercisers who really don't know their own body?

"What is my point of exhaustion? What is anaerobic threshold?"

Anaerobic threshold is the point when your body shifts from aerobic (steady) states of exercise to anaerobic (gasping) states. It is also where your muscles start to hurt from excess lactic acid, produced by physical stress. Essentially, the point of exhaustion or breathlessness is the point where you can no longer carry on a conversation (because you are out of breath). If you can't carry on a conversation while you are exercising, then you have exceeded your anaerobic threshold, and this can be dangerous.

Always give yourself the "talk test" while exercising!

Do not be discouraged if you cannot walk and talk at the same time. This will come with time (and miles walked!). In the second half of this book, we will discuss how to start a walking and/or exercise program that you can build on during your pregnancy. As you build endurance, you will also build a higher anaerobic threshold. Be patient!

So, what is the reasonable heart rate??

It's hard to know what is "reasonable" if you've never tested yourself before. Here is why the workout journal is so important. Workout as you normally would but be sure to stop periodically throughout the workout and test your heart rate. If you cross train, walking one day and doing circuit training the next – test your heart rate with every different activity. Write down these bpm (heart beats per minute) with a description of what you were doing. It is important to measure your resting state so that you can have a better idea of how hard you are actually working.

There are a number of excellent heart monitors on the market that do the work for you, keeping an accurate measure of your bpm. Or, simply do it the old fashioned way. Applying pressure to any of the major arteries that are close to the surface. The two most popular ways to measure your pulse rate is the wrist (radial artery) and the neck (carotid artery).

- ■ Before even getting out of bed, take your heart rate. Of course, if the super sonic alarm clock clangs overhead, making your heart pound, give yourself a few more moments to relax before testing yourself.

- After you've located your pulse, use the second hand on the clock and begin counting the number of heart beats for exactly one minute. You can use a digital clock but it is best to use the second hand on a watch or clock.
- At one minute, stop counting. This is your resting state. The average healthy woman has a rate of 75 bpm – but everyone is different.
- Write down this resting state measurement in your journal and continue to do this for several days to get a better idea of what is your average resting state.

The next question is, "How intensely do you work out?" This is your training heart rate and very important in determining what your "reasonable" workout heart rate can or should be. You will need to take your pulse again while exercising. As you did before:

- When you are fully into your training routine (an aerobic class, spinning, Stairmaster, walking…), stop periodically to check your rate heart/pulse.
- Write down the number of bpm.
- Repeat this for the next several exercise days and measure your results against the other workouts.
- If you are too tired to count, here's a quick way to count. Pressing against your carotid artery, count the bpm for a full six seconds – then multiply by ten.

Whether you are a seasoned athlete or a beginner to the exercise game, you should workout at the intensity between 50 – 85 percent. As a rule, your work efforts should be:

Beginner or low fitness level . . .50% - 60%
Average fitness level . . . . 60% - 70%
High fitness level . . . . 75% - 85%

Ahh. So, the final question is, how do you determine what a reasonable heart rate is for you while exercising? The more you exercise, the harder your body works. And in theory, that sounds about right. But we need to take a few things into consideration. If you're strolling along, talking on your cell phone as you walk, this is not exercise. This is strolling along, talking on your cell phone.

On the flip side, this does not mean you have to jump on the treadmill set at 20 miles per hour and full out sprint. There is a happy medium.

There is a basic formula to follow while exercising. Using the theory that your maximum heart rate is 220 beats per minute, minus your age. The average intensity level (performance activity) is at 65 percent. An elite athlete should be working at 75 to 85 percent.

Multiply your work at 65 percent from your maximum bpm (220) minus your age.

Akkk! What are you talking about?!?
To make it easier, look at the equation:

220 – (your age) and multiply by 0.65 = your target heart rate.
So, if you are 20, 25, 30, 35, 40, or 45 here is your average heart rate:

220 – 20 x .65 =   130
220 - 25 x. 65 =   127
220 - 30 x .65 = 124
220 – 35 x .65 =   120
220 - 40 x .65 =   117

Heart Rate vs. Common Sense

Throughout the book, I mention that it is important to stop if something doesn't "feel right." There are times that getting a good pulse rate seems impossible. The Borg Scale offers another measuring method – called Ratings of Perceived Exertion. The measure focuses on how you feel while working out as opposed to what your pulse rate or heart monitor reads. Often times, pregnant women can be difficult to properly measure so we ask that you pay special attention to how you feel.

It's suggested that you rate how you feel (both physically and emotionally) on a scale of 0 – 10 while working out. If you find you are between a 4 and 5 on the RPE scale, this is a good indicator that you have a good workout program and know that you are working within a reasonable heart rate in terms of intensity level. Once again, I strongly urge you to record how you feel after each workout in your journal:

0 . . . . .Nothing at all
0.5 . . . Very, very weak
1 . . . . .Very weak
2 . . . . .Weak
3 . . . . .Moderate
4 . . . . .Somewhat strong
5 . . . . .Strong
6
7 . . . . .Very strong
8
9
10 . . . .Very, very strong (Maximal)

For the more elite athlete:

Question:
My wife and I are trying to conceive. My wife is very fit right now as she runs and plays sports like soccer regularly. Given that we are trying (i.e. she might be pregnant, she might not be, who knows), my question is whether or not she should be playing in a weekend long tournament... is this much exercise too much if she we just conceived? Does the rule-of-thumb of a heart rate below 140 still apply? Thanks for the advice.

Answer:
We really watch the standard 140 bpm for women who have never really worked out or are more weekend warriors. Your wife, however, is in good shape and exercises regularly.

Of course, this is where I need to say that she should see her doctor/OB/GYN to be cleared to play soccer and continue with her athletic endeavors. There may be other medical conditions that we are unaware of so it is always safe to speak first with the doctor.

Having said this, because she is in shape (again, check first with doctors) she can go beyond the 140 bpm. I'm hoping she is a defender -- less running than the midfielder. When she sprints for the ball or down the field, her heart rate will spike. The important thing to focus on is how long does her heart rate stay elevated. Studies performed on sprint intervals allow for athletes to have a spiked heart rate, rest, spike, rest ... and so on. This would work well with her soccer playing. But if she is running the majority of the game, she needs to request more subbing or to be placed in the backfield. She and her coach need to limit her sprint intervals.

We also want to watch is her inner core temperature. Because I do not know where you live and what the current temperatures are or if it's indoor soccer -- I'll cover all the bases.
Whether it's indoor or outdoor with cooler temperatures -- both more ideal -- you will need to watch her inner core temperature.

What is it? Okay... now, steady, man. Don't get grossed out. As a soon-to-be-daddy, you better start getting used to this kind of stuff. Your baby has no way to sweat, thus, no way to cool him/herself. So, as your wife's inner core temperature rises, so will the little oven your baby is in.

A HUGE mistake women make is thinking they can simply 'feel' how hot they are. But wind, cooler temperatures, drinking water, halftime, even genetics can make it difficult for a woman to really gauge how hot she is. The only tried and true way is to use a rectal thermometer to be sure that her temperature does not rise above 101 degree F.

Communicate with her coach, let him/her know that your wife is pregnant and that she will need to be pulled from the field (if she is doing a lot of running or even if she's not running a lot but it is hot outside) so that she can run to the bathroom and check her inner core temperature.

She can also do this at half-time. When I am working out a pregnant client with more intense cardio, the general rule is every 20 minute -- check temp.

If she is playing outside and you are in hotter temperatures -- be smart. Watch the level of play time, have water-soaked rags (in ice water) for her to put on her head/around her neck, be sure she is drinking a lot of water and monitor the running time while she's on the field. Again, have her check her temp every 20 minutes for safety. If her temperature is at or near 101 degree F -- it's time to bench her.

Finally, there is one more issue. Body contact. This must be your judgment call. Some games can become quite physical. While your baby is very well protected, the last thing your wife needs is a 180-pound forward barreling down the line, slamming your wife into the ground in the greater quest of a goal. It is something that must be considered.

1. Doctor permission.
2. Buy and use rectal thermometer -- every 20 minutes.
3. Stay hydrated -- this doesn't mean just during soccer. During this period in her life -- she does not need to be drinking caffeinated coffee or colas. They will naturally dehydrate her (I can also list for you the other problems associated with caffeine during pregnancy).

4. Sit in the shade on breaks
5. Do not run the entire games. She can sprint but needs to be able to bring her heart rate down after a sprint.

In other words -- be smart. With safety guidelines in place, she should be able to play.

On a final note, you must know that her body will change as the pregnancy progresses. Soccer is such a physical sport, I want to caution you about how her joints as they will be more susceptible to injury in the latter half of her second trimester. As her body grows, her joints will loosen and ligaments will soften in preparation of labor and delivery. Cutting back and forth, dribbling the ball, faking people out may be too much on her frame. Again, have open dialogue about how she feels during and after the game. On a personal note, I would be too nervous about aggressive players on the other team. As you will later read, there are many outside factors in sports/training that cannot be controlled. When this occurs, I advise stepping away …

6. Check the Weather

As much as I caution about proper foot wear and sports bras, you also need to be aware of current weather conditions. The most obvious is heat. When asked "can I do ..." questions about sport-related activities that are outdoors, my first concern is typically about the heat. But there is dangerously little mention of air quality.

A 2004 scientific study (by Johns Hopkins and Yale Universities) found that changes in ground-level ozone were significantly associated with an increase in deaths in many U.S. cities. The risk of death was slightly higher for people with respiratory (lung) or cardiovascular (heart) problems. Experts have also become more concerned about the levels of mercury and other hazardous materials being released into our atmosphere. While environmentalists continue their fight for clean air and healthier babies, big business has been given a free pass on far too many instances. As an example, in 2003, Representative Joe Barton (R-TX), acting as chairman of the powerful House Energy and Commerce Committee, which handles legislation affecting energy, air quality, the environment, and hazardous materials, pushed through policies that allow Ellis County factories (factories which gave thousands of dollars to his re-election campaign) to have lesser environmental requirements -- meaning they are allowed to pollute more and not get in trouble for it. His explanation? "No one ever died of ozone inhalation?"

Why should you care?
Not only should you care for your own health as you begin a new exercise program or continue with your daily jogs and bike rides, but you are now a mother. This earth belongs to your baby. What you breathe does affect your baby. Ground-level ozone is an air pollutant formed by motor vehicle exhaust, industrial emissions, gasoline vapors, and chemical solvents mixing with naturally-occurring gases, NOx and VOC. When these chemicals and gases mix in sunlight and hot weather, the result is harmful pollution, known as "bad" ozone.

Question:
"I'm really worried about pollution. My husband tells me I'm just being paranoid but I breathe so heavily and I can't help but worry about what this does to our baby. Should I be worried?"

Answer:
Worried? Of course! But should this stop you from working out? No. You can make better decisions before you step outside and you can also be proactive in your own community. Remember that being healthy is just one way of being a role model to your child. In addition to teaching your baby about healthy eating and working out, you can also demand cleaner/better air and water for your family and community.

Question:

"What will pollution do to my baby?"

Answer:

How does ground-level ozone pollution affect human health? This is a great question! Low levels of ground-level ozone pollution can cause inflammation and irritation of the lungs, particularly during physical activity. This can cause shortness of breath, coughing, and throat irritation. Breathing ozone pollution can trigger asthma attacks. Exposure to high levels of ozone pollution can inflame and damage the lining of the lungs, decreasing the lungs' ability to function. And recent studies suggest that ozone doesn't just aggravate asthma; it may cause asthma. In fact, one out of every three people is at higher risk for ozone-related health effects -- including children, anyone with heart or lung disease, and adults who work or exercise outdoors.

Despite foolish remarks like "no one ever died of ozone inhalation," the truth is that many people have become very sick (even died) as a result of exposure to ground-level ozone pollution.

Pay attention to what kind of weather you are having. If it is 100 degrees outside or the air quality is very poor, do not exercise outside. You can check the quality of air in your area by logging on to the Environmental Protection Agency (EPA) site at www.airnow.gov for a national breakdown of weather and air conditions.

Question:
"The day (or air quality) is color-coded. What do they mean?"

Answer:

GREEN: No negative health impacts are expected at this stage. A green day is a good day to go for a walk, a jog, or a hike. It's a good day to play outside.

YELLOW: Unusually sensitive people -- such as people with asthma, bronchitis, other upper respiratory problems, or allergies -- need to be cautious about spending too much time outdoors or being too active.

ORANGE: This level is unhealthy for children or adults with respiratory diseases. These people should not be active outdoors on orange days, and they should avoid prolonged physical exertion.

RED: Level red is considered unhealthy for everyone, and outdoor activities such as walking, hiking, running, playing, or even riding bikes should be avoided.

PURPLE: This hazardous level is considered quite dangerous to everyone, and outdoor activity should be limited. People are discouraged from mowing lawns, raking leaves, or gardening on red and purple days. These activities should be postponed until a healthier day.

7. Your Team

Your team has not changed. Be sure to stay in contact with your medical team and lay out your long-term plans for your trainer and training buddy.

Chapter Five
What's My Problem?

A group of women sit in a circle, stretching and commiserating after a tough kickboxing class. In total, we are seventeen. We are tall, short, black, white, young, older, lean, and heavyset. We are nurses, doctors, teachers, engineers, homemakers, administrators, business owners, and a physicist. Among the group are former athletes in soccer, track and field, basketball, and swimming. It's a group of women who manage corporate accounts, deadlines, life and death. In all aspects of their lives, they are organized and in control. Yet the topic of the evening is of anything but. "Why can't I lose weight?" "Why can't I stop myself from eating so much?" "Why am I so tired all the time?"

Women around the world face tougher challenges than our male counterparts simply because of our genetic makeup. This is life. Now add to this list women who are suddenly pregnant. Raging hormones do not help insecurities of weight gain or loss, how to workout, and how life will change after the baby is born. While exercise and eating habits will certainly improve matters, they are not the end-all to all problems or emotional set-backs. There are also physical explanations to fatigue and weight issues.

1. The Hormonal Effect

Congratulations! You're pregnant. Now, step aside while the most amazing construction begins to take place. Your body is busily making major (hormonal) changes to prepare for a baby in the next 37 weeks. The glands of your endocrine system and placenta are under serious hormonal construction. Your blood volume will increase, triggering all kinds of reactions from headache to heartburn. The good news is …this is all normal. The bad news is … this is all normal.

1. **Morning Sickness**: It is more common than not to feel nauseous in the beginning of your pregnancy, including vomiting and major food aversions. Suddenly, you may have a bionic nose – able to smell a peanut from fifty feet away. Typically, these feelings will go away by the second trimester. What can help? Exercise, staying properly hydrated, rest, and bland carbohydrates such as crackers or dry toast. Focus on smaller meals throughout the day.

   *Ginger is believed to help fight morning sickness.

2. **Mood swings**: Influx of hormones can trigger feelings of anxiety, distress, and full-out crabbiness. When and where these mood swings will attack, no one knows. But we do know that exercise, a proper diet, proper sleep, and a support team can help! While you should take comfort in knowing this is normal, if you have feelings of despair, or have
thoughts of hurting yourself, please speak to your doctor right away! This DOES NOT mean you are a bad mother, a bad person, an unstable person. This means you need to speak to someone about the hormonal surges that are potentially harming you and your baby. Remember that a GOOD mother will always seek help.

3. **Constipation & Heartburn**
The increase of the hormone progesterone slows your digestive track at the same time your bowels are naturally hardened (dehydrated) as your colon absorbs more water. Otherwise soft stools become more difficult to move as they harden, thus the feeling of constipation. And, another reminder why you need to drink more water.
*Do not take a laxative. If this uncomfortable feeling persists, talk to your doctor about your options.
Heartburn, like constipation, is often triggered by the pregnancy hormones. It is a common side effect of pregnancy, caused by the backward flow of stomach acids into the esophagus, the tube that carries food from your mouth to your stomach. Smaller and more frequent meals, eating slowly (see Chapter 3: Ten Rules for the Table), and skip the fried foods. Coffee and colas often trigger heartburn as does chocolate (sorry!), garlic, and onions
*If the sensation persists, do not take antacids or other medications without first speaking to your OB/GYN.

2. Fatty Liver

As terrible as it sounds, it is one of the biggest problems Americans face today. Americans have fatty livers. While we've long known that the liver is the vital organ for ridding toxins in our bodies, little attention has been paid to how the liver processes or stores fat. In fact, one of the best explanations I've ever heard/read on the importance of the liver came from author and researcher Dr. Ann Louis Gittleman (The Fat Flush Plan, McGraw-Hill, New York, 2002) when she described, "The liver metabolizes not only fats but also carbohydrates and proteins for use in your body." But one sure sign that your liver has stopped processing fat and has begun storing it occurs when you've begun to 'store' fat at your waistline. "You may have what is commonly called a "fatty liver."

While storing fat at your waistline is not a concern during pregnancy, I am most concerned about the long-term effects of the fatty liver. How your body processes fat, how you sleep, feel, digest food, exercise, and otherwise live your life are all connected to the overall health of your liver. It is exactly that important.

Your liver may have something to do with why you feel fatigued, achy, and disconnected. Not surprisingly, there are many other medical fallouts from the fatty liver such as depression, high blood pressure, higher cholesterol, indigestion, heartburn, even skin rashes and cellulite.

Again, talk to a nutritionist to determine how you can change to a healthier lifestyle for you, your baby, and your future.

3. Anemia: Fatigue and Dizziness

Question:
"I'm exhausted all the time. I know my husband thinks I'm just being a baby but it's not that. What's wrong with me?"

Answer:
There could be a number of medical explanations for this and I suggest you see your doctor as I do not know your medical history. However, there is an equally strong likelihood that you are anemic and do not even know it.

Anemia is often called "tired blood." It is a condition in which not enough red blood cells can carry a sufficient amount of oxygen to your tissues, thus making you feel tired and weak. Red blood cells contain hemoglobin — a red, iron-rich protein that gives blood its red color. Hemoglobin enables red blood cells to carry oxygen from your lungs to all parts of your body, and to carry carbon dioxide from other parts of the body to the lungs so that it can be exhaled. The condition of anemia, in which not enough red blood cells can carry oxygen to your tissues, causes you to feel tired and weak.

It is estimated that almost 4 million Americans are anemic. Of course, there is a wide variation of anemia, ranging from mild to severe. Because of this, it is not usually until a woman gets pregnant that she learns she is or has been boarder line anemic.

This is called iron deficiency anemia and easily treated. It is believed that about one in five women and half of pregnant women are anemic in the United States. The cause is a shortage of iron in your body and without an adequate amount your body simply cannot produce enough hemoglobin for red blood cells. In pregnant women, a growing fetus can deplete the mother's store of iron, leading to iron deficiency anemia.

This is a topic I am all too familiar with. I am strong, active, and eat well (okay, except for that whole sitting in the fridge eating Smuckers and chocolate syrup thing), but while pregnant, I become quite anemic. As a teenager, I was once denied from giving blood because my iron count was too low but I'd believed that was a one-time deal. Then, suddenly, in my first pregnancy, I suffered my first bout – experiencing dizziness and disorientation so severe that I could not speak properly and was unable to turn a doorknob. Untreated, I was continuously light-headed. But by taking an iron supplement, I was healthy – and still seeking chocolate. If you believe you may be anemic, make an appointment and speak with your physician before self-medicating.

Dizziness or fainting

Despite what you see in the movies, most pregnant women don't go around passing out simply because they are pregnant. However, it is not common to become so light-headed that you might feel faint. As a result of your under-construction pregnancy state, there may be a dramatic dilation of the blood vessels of your body. During the first and even second trimester of your pregnancy, however, your blood volume may not have expanded enough, causing an almost void effect. As a result, you may suffer from lower blood pressure. Hypoglycemia (low blood sugar) and/or anemia (low red blood cell count) may occur. Of course, you need to speak with your physician right away. But you can also   eat more iron-enriched foods such as bean, red meat, green leafy vegetables and dried fruits. Be sure to properly hydrate yourself and work with a trainer – exercising to ensure good blood circulation.

Fatigue

Sometimes you're just tired. There is no mystery here. In your first trimester, there is a great and sudden demand on your body, including your circulatory system. Your body must produce extra blood to properly carry oxygen and nutrients to the fetus. As a result, your heart works harder and faster, and your body produces higher levels of progesterone, which tends to make you sleepy. If you are feeling sleepier – make sure you get what your body is asking for. Again, this isn't the time to "be tough." Take the extra naps when you can. You're under serious construction!

*Don't think you need a nutritionist?? Here's another reason to talk to someone about your food journal: Did you know that dark-skinned berries such as blackberries or purple grapes have antibodies that can actively block iron? Women with anemia are often surprised to learn their 'healthy' diet is causing more problems than not with anemia.

4. High Blood Pressure

Let's get this straight from the get-go: A woman who is diagnosed with chronic high blood pressure should not engage in a rigid or strenuous exercise routine during pregnancy because the risk to the baby's blood supply is too great.

If you are diagnosed with chronic high blood pressure, you must have an open dialogue with your physician and OB/GYN about your desire to exercise and whatever long-term goals you have.

You may be pleasantly surprised to learn that your doctor(s) have a plan for you. This would and should include a trainer and nutritionist. But the most important thing here is that you must have medical permission to continue.

To explain your condition in easy terms, the opening of blood vessels in the first trimester of your pregnancy can suddenly lower your blood pressure. Many times, a woman will not realize she had chronic high blood pressure until the latter half of her pregnancy. What is a concern, however, is many women decide to stop taking medication as their blood pressure lowers. Do not play doctor. Because of your condition, you must keep in constant contact with your physicians and let them decide how you should or shouldn't be medicated.

Medications such as methyldopa are considered to be very effective and safe for both momma and baby but should be monitored by your physician. If, medicated or not, your doctor prescribes exercise, be sure to keep a detailed journal for your Team Baby to review.

5. Thyroid

The thyroid is a gland located in front of the windpipe in the neck that makes hormones that help control the workings of many of the body's organs. In some instances, however, a woman's thyroid produces too much of the hormone (called hyperthyroidism), while others have too little (called hypothyroidism). These disorders can create a risk for both mother and baby. For this reason, it is so important to keep your regular appointments with your OB/GYN as many thyroid problems do not appear until a woman is pregnant or soon after delivery.

Remember that it is important to listen to your body. Some of the symptoms of hypothyroidism are fatigue, weight gain, disorientation, muscle and joint aches, an enlarged thyroid (goiter), feeling cold, constipation, slow heart rate and obvious hair loss.

Symptoms of hyperthyroidism are anxiety, irritability, weight loss, rapid heart beat, feeling warm, frequent stools, and/or goiters but you must know that these symptoms can also be associated with other medical problems so do not be misled. Make an appointment to meet and discuss your complaints/worries with your doctor. The good news is that with proper treatment, you should be able to have a healthy, happy pregnancy. Talk to you doctor about an exercise program and recommended nutrition plan. Again, do not begin exercise until you have devised a plan with your medical team.

6. Hypoglycemia

<u>Question</u>:
"All I keep hearing is to get control of my problem before I get pregnant. But I'm already pregnant. What am I supposed to do now?"

Answer:
You're right. For obvious reasons, your physician and OB/GYN would like to see your hypoglycemia under control as it greatly reduces the risks of miscarriages, birth defects, and complications during labor and delivery. Those are some pretty scary thoughts. These are the primary concerns in the first trimester.

During your second trimester, if untreated, there is concern about your baby growing too large (macrosomia). This condition affects approximately 40 percent of babies born to diabetic mothers.

This is where Team Baby comes in. You must speak with your OB/GYN and a nutritionist about heavy glucose levels as your pregnancy moves along. Because your body is constantly changing and because hormonal changes may increase your resistance to insulin you can't guess what or how to eat. To that, women with Type 2 diabetes or previous gestational diabetes may need to inject the hormone during pregnancy.

- Note that oral diabetes medications can cause birth defects, so women using them should switch to insulin while pregnant.

As with many other medical conditions, you must consult your physician, OB/GYN and dietitian – Team Baby – before you begin to exercise. Again, it would be ideal to work with Team Baby before there is a baby but once you are pregnant, you must become proactive!

7. Fertility and Miscarriages

<u>Question:</u>
My husband and I are trying to conceive, and we just moved across the country to a new house. We want to know if there is any danger to a possible pregnancy from me lifting boxes as we unpack. I would estimate that most boxes weigh 30 pounds, maybe 40. That's all I can lift! I know moderate exercise is a good thing for me, before and during pregnancy, and I know how to lift properly, but I want to make sure about any risks to dislodging the pregnancy from lifting things specifically.

Answer:

This is a tough question. For many women, lifting 30-pounds would be very easy while it could be challenging -- too challenging – for others. Ideally, if you are an active person who lifts weights (moderately), do not have any other medical issue I don't know about (hypertension, diabetes, anemia …etc), and are in fact lifting properly, there should be no reason to worry about lifting 30 lbs boxes. But again, the real question is how much can you lift when you're not pregnant? The important thing is that as an active, in-shape person, you lift what you could/would have pre-pregnant.

If you've been a relatively sedentary person, have not lifted weights, are unsure about how much you can lift, and have not spoken with your doctor, I would not advise moving box after box. You can certainly be of great help by packing and unpacking the boxes without moving them.

Another concern is your level of exhaustion, heat and physical strain.

To clarify, many people lose track of time while they are moving and do not properly hydrate themselves. And no, drinking a coke doesn't count! By working long hours packing and hauling, your body needs to be replenished with water. The water will keep you hydrates and allow you to stay cool. We often forget and don't realize how hot we've become. As you become more tired, you will lose the proper form to lift and move boxes – so take plenty of breaks.

Question:

"We have been trying to conceive for three years. I have an extremely irregular cycle which the doctor is blaming on my weight. I think stress is a factor. That is what I am working on. My fertility specialist is recommending weight loss. What is the best way to go about this and should I be taking vitamins or doing anything else to help?"

Answer:

There are a number of factors that may increase infertility and you just hit on two of them: weight and stress. But I promise you, stress outweighs weight (no pun intended). You need to do a life change that will help you conceive. Adopt an exercise routine. Yes, studies have shown that women who work out regularly are better able to conceive.

Before you begin, you must see your physician. Once you have a medical permission to exercise, make five important steps:

1. Begin a food journal. Start watching and recording what you eat.
2. Increase your water intake, lay off the caffeine and sugar drinks.
3. Contact a trainer or join a women's gym, such as Curves, where you are guided through a circuit training program. I suggest a women's gym because it tends to be more low-key and stress-free!
4. Begin taking vitamins. Too many women wait until after they are pregnant to take a prenatal vitamin. Most likely, your body can benefit from the nutrients now.

5. Find a nutritionist to take a look (after one week) at your food journal. Sit down and discuss what changes you need to make and what changes you are realistically willing to take.

Once you've begun this routine, the increase of your body's blood flow and metabolism will kick in, endorphins (natural hormones) will step up, sending signals to your brain – reeeellllaaaaxxxxx!

By taking care of your body naturally and feeling as though you have some kind of 'wellness' game plan, thereby reducing stress, you will greatly increase your chances of getting pregnant while getting healthy. Good luck!

Question:

Hi. I am 30-year old woman who is very physically active. I run about 8-10 miles a day and take a Pilates class once a week. My husband and I are looking to start trying to get pregnant soon and I would like to know if I need to decrease my work out in order to conceive? And by how much is reasonable? I started the Pilates so that I can integrate something less intense than running but don't know how soon I need to cut back the running to conceive.

Answer:

Elite athletes and marathon runners get pregnant all the time. The key here is heat. I don't know where you live, but running over 4 miles really drives up the inner core temperature. As you run, your inner core temp gets higher and higher. It has been argued that this makes conception more difficult and many scientists believe that elite athletes will abort without even knowing they were ever pregnant due to intense training. However, the bulk of these athletes are singly focused on better times, better splits, more grueling routes. They are not thinking about pregnancy.

I was training for the US bobsled team, running distances and sprints, lifting very heavy weights and doing intense plyometircs when I got pregnant. But here's the thing... I was planning a pregnancy. Not only was I able to train as hard as my teammates – I believe I was more focused BECAUSE I was so centered on my pregnancy. In fact – and I mention this only to illustrate the point that one does not have to give up elite sport – I won the US Nationals while four months pregnant.

But – I was careful. I did not run in the heat. I checked my inner core temperature with a rectal thermometer. I know. It's disgusting but it ensured safety at all times. Because your baby's temp is one degree Celsius higher than your own temperature and your baby does NOT have any sweating mechanism, it is essential that you do not allow your own body temperature to exceed 101 degrees. You can't simply "feel" how hot you are or can't take oral/ear temperature because you must know your inner temp. – the rectal thermometer is needed. So, I would run behind bleachers, behind bushes, into bathrooms every 20-25 minutes when I was working cardio.

84

I made sure to stay hydrated and on longer runs – have water brought to me. This is a royal pain but you do what you have to do to ensure safety.

Also, if you are a smaller person – lower body fat – your chances of conceiving will be a little harder statistically speaking. Again, this might be a reason to back off the higher miles for a while. Do you have to stop running?? No. But you might want to knock things down to 4-5 miles for a bit and try a different kind of aerobics class.

But first, you must see your doctor. While you are happy running 8-10 mile a day (wow!), we don't know your medical history. It's important that your personal physician is on board with your running and Pilates, that both agree you are able to do this medically speaking and have a candid conversation about your desire to become pregnant. The instant you believe you are pregnant, see your OB/GYN. You should be warned that many OB/GYN's still shy away from a woman working out while pregnant. Given the information you've provided, I doubt there should be any problems, but listen to your medical team. Once you've become pregnant, let us know and we'll discuss your pregnancy workout routine.

It's Not Just You!

That's right, baby. Daddy has a bigger role than you realize. His use of nicotine and caffeine may directly affect his sperm count, as can the amount of time he sits on the bicycle. Prolonged hours on the bike can damage sperm count due to the constant pressure on the seat. Contact sports can lead to injury to the testicles can also cause sperm production. Even use of a lap top (sitting on his lap) can affect sperm count.

Relax

The theme here, as you've read, is stress. Women of all ages, size, and backgrounds worry about .. well, they worry. I'm too heavy, I'm too thin. I am too active or not active enough. As you read along, it is my hope that you will begin a food/drink/vitamin journal even before you've finished the book. You may begin life changes today that may indeed help start your family.

If you are considered a high-risk with your doctor, the rules are still the same. Talk to your medical team about what it is you want. Lose weight? Better health? Gain weight? How does this play into trying to conceive? Talk to you doctor about exercise and diet. Contact a trainer and nutritionist to safely set you on course.

Remember that as you begin to feel that you are in control of your life, great things may happen.

Question:
"I've heard that too much exercise can cause a miscarriage!"

Answer:

It was once believed that exercise could cause your membranes to rupture, causing spontaneous pre-mature labor and/or miscarriage. Today, we know better. In fact, for women who are already reasonably active (and with your doctor's permission, of course), you can safely continue your exercise during pregnancy.

So, the question is, what is too much exercise? You must use common sense. Working to exhaustion, lifting heavy weights, and doing anything you are unaccustomed to is a bad idea. But if you continue to work out as you have, or begin a safe walking program and exercise throughout, you actually have a better chance of a healthier, safer pregnancy.

Play it smart. Play is safe. If you have a history of early labors, hypertension, thyroid, heart or lung disease, or any medical condition that has been red-flagged by your OB/GYN and personal physician, you MUST follow doctor's orders. In these cases, do not take the word of an optimistic trainer. Trainer and doctor must be on board together.

If you have a history of bleeding or spotting, you must talk to your doctor about this. Being scared or nervous but saying nothing is a dangerous course. Be open and honest with members of Team Baby at all times.

8. Vitamins – Or the Lack Thereof

Question:

"I don't take any vitamins and I'm four months pregnant. I tried but they make me really sick to my stomach. Is that okay?"

Answer:

No. You really need to properly nourish your body. Because you have increased demands on your body, because your body requires almost twice as much protein, because your body's immune system will often be taxed, you need to be taking a prenatal vitamin.

Besides protein, you need iron to build blood cells (and prevent anemia), zinc to create a healthy fetus, calcium for your bones (and teeth) as the baby will naturally deplete your stores, taking what he or she needs. Your baby will also need folic acid to prevent premature births and birth defects.

Because prenatal vitamins can often cause nausea, it is a good idea to take the prenatal vitamin before going to bed. You will sleep through the waves of nausea you might otherwise experience. Also, because you are sleeping, thus using the bathroom less often (although not by much), your body is less likely to flush the vitamin and it's benefits through your body. You will better absorb the nutrients!

And if you're looking for another reason to take vitamins, how about this? Vitamins A, C, and E help insulin action and enable your body to better regulate glucose. In other words, it helps your metabolism.

9. Your Team

You should not wait to create your Team Baby team until after you are pregnant. I cannot count the number of questions in which a question or comment was made regarding the lack of support a woman feels from friends and family as she contemplates motherhood. Whether it's because of economical, medical, or personal reasons, this is a huge, life-altering time in your life. You must have all the support you can get. You need to have a medical team that is open and honest with you, ready to work with whatever medical issues you have. You need to have a trainer who can create a safe yet challenging exercise routine that will offer you all the benefits of being a fit mother. You should have a nutritionist who can assess your eating and drinking habits and help you make the right moves. You need to have a training buddy who will entertain, engage, encourage and inspire you.

If you are trying to get pregnant, you must believe that the changes you are making have great purpose, with even better outcomes. And once you are pregnant, you should have a team that will remind you that as a mother, you are expected to be as strong of a role model as you can possibly be.

Everyone needs a Team Baby.

Chapter Six
Already an Athlete??

Many women wrestle with the word 'athlete.' We're conditioned to think of an athlete as someone who plays a sport professionally. Because they are simply dedicated to their gym or fitness routine, they don't think the word 'athlete' applies. But would you consider a professional golfer or bowler an athlete? Or, to rephrase, do they have the athlete's body?

If you are committed to a routine, if you consider what and how you eat as it will affect your body and your workouts, you ARE an athlete. It's a label you should wear with honor and not worry that you will have to give it up simply because you are pregnant.

1. What Will the Neighbors Say?

"Wow! Finally, someone who can say more than "don't get overheated" and "check with your doctor" about prenatal fitness! It is great to read your answers to other questions on your website, especially the day after my doctor told me I should stop running completely because it shakes the baby too much."

I hear this a lot. Because there are so many fitness trainers and physicians who have not yet taken the time to learn about female athletes and their pregnancies, many misconceptions still exist.

While I trained extensively for the U.S. bobsled team, I had noticed (through detailed journaling) that my baby always seemed very quiet during exercise and, in turn, while I was trying to rest or sleep, her own aerobics routine began. Out of sheer sleep-deprived frustration, I once asked Dr. Clapp about Katie's romper womb-aerobics. Often times, babies of athlete moms are lulled into sleep by the mother's activities. Only when I was still did she become active. I took this as a positive sign that even in utero, babies like exercise.

Just because you are pregnant, does not mean you have to stop exercise. As you will continue to read, the benefits to both mother and baby are far reaching.

Question:
"I want to keep working out but I get so many stares or comments in the gym. Should I quit? Am I doing too much as I am almost eight months pregnant?"

Answer:
Only you can answer these next questions:

1. Do your doctor and OB/GYN know what you are doing? Or, are you medically cleared to exercise? At-risk moms should be taking it easy at this stage in the pregnancy. I want to be sure that not only do you have medical clearance but your doctors know exactly what you are doing. If you are working out on the stationary bike, for example, that's fine. But if you're running suicides in the basketball court, well…. There may be a very good reason why people are staring at you. (By the way, if that's what you're doing … knock it off!!)

2. Are you working within a safety zone? That is, not keeping your heart rate elevated for too long, not allowing yourself to get too hot, and checking your inner core temperature?

3. Are you working out for you rather than other people? (Read the following segment: "It's Not a Contest.") It is important that you not show off, proving how strong you are while others watch (and judge). You should be working out for comfort, enjoying the workout, feeling the good that it is doing, rather than draining yourself.

If you are doing all of these things, then you must not worry what others think. For the most part, they all probably still believe a pregnant woman should not be working out at all. You know what is best for you. Don't worry about anyone else but you and baby.

2. Acclimated Muscles

You've heard this term quite a few times in the answers regarding continued exercise while pregnant. So, what does this mean?

Question:
"I am four to five week pregnant and I'm registered to run a 4 mile run very soon. I have been running all my life and wanted some advice about if I can continue to run. I'm in good shape and love the exercise!"

Answer:
You are in perfect form to run. As you have been in training "all your life," this four-mile run should be a jog in the park! But before you tie up those laces, let's get a few things clear:

1. You need to be sure that you are medically clear to exercise.
2. Be sure that you are properly hydrated.
3. Consider the heat index. Most mothers-to-be focus on heart rate but you need to know what your inner core temperature is. By taking trial runs, stopping to

take your inner core temperature half-way through the course, you can and will know that your inner core temperature is in the safety zone by race day.

4. Weather. If it is cool outside on race day and you know what your inner core temperature has been through training (and temperature taking!), you should be good to go. However, if it is hot outside – you need to consider how the heat outside will affect your own inner core temperature.

5. During your trial runs, do check your heart rate. As a lifelong runner, your body is acclimated to such runs and you will easily find your comfort zone while you run. But if you are struggling on hills, steep inclines or trying to make a specific time, I want you to be aware of an elevated heart rate – and sustained elevated heart rate. No race is worth overheating or overloading yourself. Play it safe.

As your pregnancy progresses, you may find that the pounding of your foot striking the surface is a little too hard on the joints and the ever-expanding tummy. Move indoors and try a treadmill or, as many runners do, bring it down to a fast walk. Remember, comfort is the key. As a lifelong athlete, you will rebound quickly.

Good luck with the race!

For this athlete, her body is acclimated to the chore of running. What concerns me most are the women who suddenly want to begin a workout routine after a lifetime of couch-sitting. For the athlete, as long as the activity is not a new one, your muscles are completely acclimated to the movements/stress of running, hiking, cycling, or whatever it is you usually do.

Many athletes worry because once they become pregnant, they are suddenly winded and tired as they never have been before. This is typical and usually occurs in the first trimester. The answer to this new situation is easy: ride it out comfortably. If you're suddenly gasping for air, bring it down, walk it off or stop the activity all together until you are able to catch your breath again.

Because you are in a new form of training – baby training – you can loosen up on the times and/or distances. Who cares? Just know that it is common.

As an athlete, however, you will read very little about this subject. When we talk about breathlessness and pregnancy, it is usually related to the last trimester when the uterus begins pushing your diaphragm toward your lungs. But because we've all been conditioned to think that pregnant women should not exercise (at least, not at certain levels) no one really discusses exercise-induced breathlessness in the first trimester.

Check your heart rate. Is it elevated? How long has it been elevated? This is why a fitness journal is so important. For elite athletes, the heart rate of 160 bpm may be as normal as eating a bowl of cereal. For others, a sudden spike in a heart rate of 160 should be your red flag to settle down, take a water break and allow your body to recover. It is essential that you know your body, your heart rate at resting state and exercising in the comfort zone, that is, when you are able to comfortably carry on a conversation. Remember the talk test? When you cannot speak normally, this is the spike (or anaerobic) rate that you need to record and be aware of. You should not stay at this rate.

Question:
"I am five weeks pregnant and was wondering if you could tell me what a safe heart rate is. I am currently working out between 140 and 170 bpm.

Also, is it safe to be wanting to do a bike ride – 1000 people in South Africa in March. I will be 3 months then. I have been training for a triathlon, a mini one in February.

Answer:
Congrats! It sounds like you are already in good shape but you must first consult your physician to be sure you are allowed to exercise. Assuming, however, you do not have any medical roadblocks and do, in fact, work out regularly, there is no reason you cannot continue to work within the 140 to 170 range.

Studies have found that elite (Olympic) athletes could and have safely worked out, heart rates exceeding well over 170 beats per minute. This is not a license to follow that same routine but to let you know that while monitored, elite athletes have safely gone beyond 170 bpm. On a personal note, I would stay where you are. Remember that these athletes have trainers and state-of-the-art equipment around them or they have already made the decision to "go for the gold." You're not willing to exchange safety for a medal, are you?

In addition, these athletes were sure not to sustain an elevated heart rate. For example, while doing sprint training, your heart rate can exceed 160 beats per minute but when you reach your peak, bring it back down. It is then important to let your heart rate go back down to the 'safety zone' of 140 to 160 beats per minute. Elite athletes wear both fetal and heart monitors when doing sprint work so they can keep a close eye on the heart range and are sure not to let it stay too high for too long.

The good news for you is that what you are doing requires slow twitch fibers (a prolonged activity) and you can/should settle into a nice, comfortable pace, keeping your heart rate at an even level. Do not set out to win the race! Simply pedal along and enjoy your company. I would like to note, however, that I do not recommend cycling outside simply because of factors you cannot control, such as other bikes crashing into you, slick roads and the chance of falling to the ground. This is the same with horseback riding and skiing. The activity itself is not as dangerous as being thrown and crashing into a tree. Please use great caution.

Finally, more important than the heart rate is your internal body temperature. You're in AFRICA! It is crucial that you pay attention to your inner core temperature. All too often, pregnant athletes do not consider how hot they become while working out and focus only on the heart rate. Because your baby has no sweating mechanism AND is one degree Celsius hotter than you/your inner core temperature, you must be conscious of how hot you become. Over the years, I have heard many ask, "Yes, but can't I just tell if I am getting too hot or not?" Not always. Many times, as you are working out, your body temperature is far hotter than you realize. Perhaps you are not sweating very much. This may not be a real indicator of how hot you are.

Whether you are running or biking, dash off to a bathroom or cluster of trees (sorry, not pretty but a must) and, using a rectal thermometer, take your inner core temp. It should not exceed 101 degree F. Be sure to drink plenty of fluids throughout your exercise. That, combined with a heart monitor and continuous check on your inner core temp, should put you on a very safe course. Still, talk to your own personal physician and explain what your exercise routine will be. And, good luck.

As you will read in Part II of the book, athletes who are acclimated to soccer, track, basketball, and weight lifting, to name a few activities, are allowed to continue so long as they've been given medical clearance. Your muscles are trained (even recreationally speaking) to move, flex, and react in a manner you are familiar with. As long as you stay with an activity you have been doing for some time, use the cautionary heat index and heart rate measures, work with your doctor and trainer, and work out for the joy of working out, you should have a great time. As always, listen to your body. It will tell you when the fun is over.

3. Check with Team Baby

Whether you are a seasoned runner, an avid hiker, a soccer referee, weekend warrior on the basketball court, or lead server in a volleyball league, do not become overconfident in your abilities. Far too often, athletes – by virtue of being athletes – feel so strong and empowered, there is little thought given to talking to a trainer, working out with a buddy, or updating a doctor on their fitness routine. But guess what? You are going to change. Your joints, weight, posture, muscles, even feet are going to change. Therefore, it is important that you continue to work with Team Baby:

1. **Your Doctor** – Stay current on your scheduled appointments. Rather than smiling and saying everything is okay, bring in a written list of what you are doing and eating, how you are feeling, and any changes you've noted that you have questions about. This includes how your workout has changed. "Well, I used to do the StairMaster but lately, I've noticed that my lower back hurts after about 20 minutes so I do the stationary bike instead." Ahhh. This is

important information that you might have otherwise blown off because now the bike feels good, right? Crisis averted. But maybe not. You need to explore why the lower back is hurting and make sure this is not a precursor to an injury.

2. **Your Trainer/Your Buddy** – Because you are an athlete, there is an inclination to NOT tell a trainer about a "weak" moment. Maybe you skipped a particular set because you were breathless but didn't want your trainer or buddy to know that you could not perform that task. Again, this is a no-no. It should be noted and questioned why you weren't able to perform a task. Was it too hard? Too heavy? This is important because as your body is changing, you need to know when too much is, in fact, too much.

3. **Your Journal** -- It's hard enough to remember all the finer details of the day without being pregnant. But now that you are pregnant, you may have noticed that you are more forgetful. Believe it or not, there is scientific evidence that while pregnant, your brain actually shrinks. Egads! While it's only a temporary condition, it explains so much . . .
Write down all the details of your workouts and nutritional intake – no matter how seemingly insignificant. This information will prove invaluable to your trainers and doctors.

4. Advise for the "Super Fit"

Question:
"There are very few articles for the very fit, big exercisers who fall pregnant. Should one cut back? How much? There are stories about Russian athletes who were made pregnant just before the Olympics as women are strongest in their first three months of pregnancy. Any news on those kinds of stories? Advice for the super-fit rather than those trying to get fit? You can't believe how little/no material there is on fitness and pregnancy in South Africa."

Answer:
I lived what you've described. While training for the US women's bobsled team, I got pregnant. At the time I was running competitive sprint times, squatting over 300 lbs, lifting, running, performing plyometrics and, in general, training like a wild woman. News of my pregnancy caused most teammates and coaches to wish me luck and show me the door. Most of the information regarding working out while pregnant was overly cautious and not even what I would have considered my warm-up. I was very nervous and didn't know what to do. Fortunately, the USOC helped turn me on to the leading researching in OB/GYN for pregnant athletes. For decades, he has been studying varying results of pregnant athletes, the most intense training being cross-country skiing and

marathon competitors. When he learned I was doing sprinting, running stadium stairs and lifting heavy weights, he was thrilled and immediately put me in his study. Because he was far away, we made special arrangements for me to travel to his laboratory and he even came (with staff) to my hometown gym. I wore fetal monitors, heart monitors, EKG leads, oxygen mask, and a rectal thermometer. Everything was monitored as I trained. (All of this is documented in my book, **Entering the Mother Zone: Balancing Self, Health, and Family** (Wish Publishing, 2000) which can be obtained through www.pregnancy.org) I learned that many of the Russian and Eastern Block Germans actually got pregnant just before the Olympics to get that hormonal rush that acts as effectively -- yet naturally -- as steroids. Most of those same athletes elected to abort shortly after competition. Shocking but true. And, that controversy continues today with other growing communist nations. As for me, when I entered the US National trials, the bet was I would come in somewhere in the middle. The last event of the competition was to push a 425 lbs sled 100 meters, scored by timing eyes. Who can push the sled the fastest? I ripped out a time that surprised even me. I felt power and energy I cannot describe. I knew I would do better than expected because I had been killing my training partners in our endurance and weight lifting tests but when I pushed off the starting blocks, everyone was yelling, "No fair! She's got TWO people pushing." It was extraordinary. Here I had been afraid I would be slow and cumbersome. I won US Nationals, was featured in **Sports Illustrated** and was named *Athlete of the Year* by the United States Olympic Committee. I was four and half months pregnant. The silver medallist? A woman named Liz Parr-Smestad who just happened to be three months pregnant.

Now, the history of the pregnant athlete is one thing. Safely applying your workout routine to your pregnant body is another matter. It is important that you consult your physician to get a clear bill of health for you and baby. Investing in a rectal thermometer is a must. It is icky to think about but may just be the most important training tool you will own.

As for your particular training routine, I would stay away from unnecessary bounding and lifting until you have talked to/worked with a trainer. You must remember that no matter how strong your body is in the first trimester, your body does change. By my fifth month, my doctor and I agreed I should stop the sprint training on the track and I worked 'sprint' training on the stationary bike. Again, I was hydrated and kept careful eye on my inner core temperature. By my seventh month, I laid off on the heavier weights as joints begin to loosen and shift. Be kind to your body, do not push too hard in the last month and have confidence in 'muscle memory.' Please do let us know what your routine is but the overall message is, you can continue doing what you are doing but be ready to adjust your routine as you grow.

5. It's Not a Contest

Question:
"What do you think of working out while pregnant? I used to ski competitively and know I can't ski while pregnant (right?) but I'm competitive. I want to stay in top shape. Can I keep on workout out?"

Answer:
Yes. No. No. Yes.

Let me break that down.

Yes, you can work out while pregnant. As long as you have medical permission, you can continue to work out. Given your athletic background and knowledge of work out, you would be safe to continue.

No. You should not ski. You are wise to step away from that activity for now. As you will read in Part II, sports specific activities, skiing is most definitely on a list of non-controlled sports.

No, you cannot stay in 'top' shape. You're pregnant. You will naturally have to step away from the more intense training during your pregnancy but that does not mean you cannot stay in great shape, continue to work on your cardio, muscles, and core strength – all things you will certainly need for labor and delivery.

Yes. By all means, take the workout program you have right now, minus the skiing, and hit the gym. But we may need to tweak a few things. Because I do not know exactly what your workout entails, you will want to work with a trainer to reevaluate your program. You can and should lift weights. However, if you are squatting heavy weights – as many competitive skiers do – you will need to adjust the weights for your ever-changing body. The idea is not to overload your back/core and legs with heavy weight. Now, you want to stay focused on flexibility, keeping your muscles viable, and good endurance.

For the most part, I am always thrilled to see a pregnant woman working out. For all the obvious health benefits (see Chapter 8, Why Even Bother?), everyone wins. But there have been times when I was distressed to see a particular pregnant woman in training. I'll give you one example.

A woman who was a five-time a week gym user was quite active in step aerobics, use of the treadmill, StairMasters, and circuit training. Already lean, she was determined to stay that way and had vowed that her pregnancy would not side-line her "too much."

As she began to show, both men and women would praise her for her commitment to working out. In class, people lovingly teased her and she was used as a measuring stick of hard work by instructors. "Come on! If she can do it ..."

Briefly, people enjoyed watching her growing belly as she came in to work out but we all soon realized this mother-to-be was trying to live up to the hype of Super

Mom. Her idea of "super" had been deluded by all the well-meaning comments in the beginning of her pregnancy.

By her third trimester, it had become such a concern that management of the gym began watching her. Instructors, trainers, even members tried to persuade her to "slow down," "take it easy," and "listen to your body."

For whatever reasons, she dug in, all the more determined to show everyone how strong she was and how well she was able to manage the workouts. What we saw was an already too-thin woman, working out to near exhaustion. Red-faced and dripping with sweat, she was clearly ignoring all the signals her body was giving.

6. I'm in Shape! Why Am I So Tired?!

"Why am I so suddenly tired all the time? I used to run five miles a day. Now I can't even run one. What gives?"

Remember that your pregnancy is only a temporary journey. You have to accept some changes, such as weight gain and fatigue. The good news is as an athlete, your group has an easier time adjusting to this change. But, as you've noted, this is not the only change. However temporary, your physical abilities and peak performances are going to change.

There is an initial peak at about three months, but after that it will gradually slide backwards until after the baby is born. This, more than weight gain and morning sickness, is the hardest thing for athletes to accept.

In 1984, while doing research at the University of Vermont, Dr. Clapp found that only 10 percent of his subjects were able to perform at pre-pregnancy workout levels throughout the pregnancy. In 1989, he later determined that his subjects' overall performance decreased approximately 10 percent in early pregnancy, then gradually to 50 percent into the third trimester.

Nausea and early-pregnancy fatigue were the cause of the initial decrease in performance, while weight gain and changing body composition were the causes for the latter part of the pregnancy. But cardiovascular fitness was maintained throughout the pregnancy, once again illustrating that one can and will stay fit through pregnancy with regular exercise.

So what does this mean for you? As your body grows and puts on more weight, your "peak" level will naturally come down a little, but that doesn't man your level of exercise intensity had to come down as well. For example, if you were running a six-minute mile pre-pregnancy, you may now be running an eight-, nine, ten-minute mile during pregnancy, but you are working just as hard – a level of intensity and the cardiovascular benefits have not gone down. You're moving more slowly because your body composition has changed, but you are still staying fit and keeping your baby healthy, which is the most important consideration. Let your body taper off naturally (as most athletes do). Listen to your body. Accept these changes as part of your – and your baby's – journey. Trying to fight this and increase or maintain your workouts is unrealistic – and potentially harmful.

Question:
"I feel strong. Really strong. Is there such a thing as too much training?"

Answer:
Yes. At a certain level of excessive exercise, blood will be diverted away from your uterus and from the baby. Training, for example, three or four hours a day may be a danger to your baby and, frankly, not something you should be willing to do.

Over the years, the doctors and athletes I have worked with/spoken to are sure that continuing the same level of exertion you were used to before pregnancy can be safe with the proper precautions. (Review Chapter Four for safety guidelines). But to push yourself beyond that point is not. While there have been many documented pregnant marathon runners, I have to wonder why an athlete would be willing to experiment with such a long, intense training program while pregnant.

A true athlete knows her own body. A true athlete also understands that through hard work, she can get her body back into top shape again. So, there is no reason to turn pregnancy into a contest.

Set small goals for yourself. The main goal is to have a healthy and happy pregnancy. But you can create smaller goals. Talk with your trainer, training buddy, and/or physician to write down realistic and healthy goals.

Remember that goals do not have to be all about physical activity. You can also strive to quit caffeine and fast food, buy more organic foods, or be more dedicated to keeping a journal.

Chapter Seven
The Couch Potato: Where Do We Go
From Here?

The very fact that you're reading this book is an excellent step forward. So, I want to tread lightly here and not scare you away from the idea that you can get in shape and improve your health. No gimmicks, no promises. The reality is, no matter what kind of shape you are in (or not), no matter what kind of physical activity you have done in the past (or not), you CAN get into shape. You can improve your overall health and happiness.

But rather than offer facts and boring scientific data, how about reading about real women, all self-described couch potatoes, who have made serious changes in their lives and are feeling the benefits?

1. The Pregnancy.org Dream Team

When the on-line non-profit organization www.pregnancy.org launched their Fitness Makeover challenge, a dream team of twelve women from around the nation were chosen. From Florida to Alaska, first-time moms to season diaper bag-toting veterans, the women were chosen from an essay they'd posted on-line, stating why they wanted to benefit from an on-line group fitness challenge.

The judges, pregnancy.org's founder Mollee Olenick, Julie Snyder and I chose women based on their determination to get healthy. Those who mentioned being a role model for their children made the A list. It was a difficult decision as we did not want to exclude anyone ready to make a life change. Therefore, the women who were ultimately chosen posted their fitness and food journals on-line so that others could follow along. The women were given the tools for great success: how-to and nutritional guides, their own personal journal for fitness and food, and light hand weights to get started. They also had nutritional and fitness expert resources on-line with an on-line "team" who were always there to chat, share, celebrate, and commiserate.

Many who were initially enthusiastic discovered that time and effort was going to be involved and dropped out. Others faded when immediate results were not seen. Alas, this is a common thread with Americans in general. Everything is fast. Fast food, one-stop shopping, instant oatmeal, call waiting, microwave cooking, and e-mails have made us impatient for anything we have to wait on or work for.

You can read how they worked out in Part III: Post-Pregnancy Workouts but it is important to note that two of the women chosen were actually pregnant at the time of the Fitness Challenge. Cyndi, a 32-year-old with a 16-month-old baby was pregnant again. She is diabetic and wanted to make sure she didn't put on too much weight while pregnant so soon after having baby #1. Beth, 30, already with a toddler, is insulin resistant, a high-risk pregnancy and also worried about her diet.

Throughout this chapter, we will discuss Cyndi and Beth, as they represent so many pregnant women. Another common theme in this book is the 'team' aspect of training. There is no better example than Cathy Bradford and her husband, Dave. Cathy was one of the "Determined Dozen" because of her fabulous attitude. In fact, she was the woman who laughed at me, stating, "I don't run unless someone is chasing me!" Between raising her children and working as a waitress at night (constantly on her feet), she had precious little time to exercise. But she did it.

By week five, she was calling my home. "I ran! I ran!" And who was right there with her? Dave. When Cathy struggled with energy or time management, Dave pushed her. The important thing to note with the workouts of the Determined Dozen was all faced challenges of some sort. Those who really wanted to make a life change dealt with the challenges and still found time to exercise.

2. "I'm Fat" and "I'm Lazy": Today's Motto

An interesting phenomenon has taken place in the last decade. Once upon a time, people would be ashamed to say, "Hey, I'm fat and lazy. That's just the way it is!" Today, as almost a reflex to our rising state of obesity, it is stated as unemotional fact. But when your own body mass, your health, and emotional attitude can actually be costing you your own life, it can't "just be the way it is."

Obesity is triggered by poor diet, poor nutrition and physical health, among other things. Following this is exhaustion, poor self-esteem, and more medical problems. Far too many people suffering with weight problems believe that it is simply too late to get into shape. I know of a woman who finally decided to battle her weight and begin a walking program. Without a training buddy, her inhaler, or a cell phone, she had an asthma attack. Her first response? "Serves me right for trying to get into shape."

Too many people view fitness and proper nutrition as a punishment. This is huge mistake number one.

Let me ask you this. If you know of a local gas station that dilutes their pumps with water, you would not go there, right? You make sure you have the tires rotated and oil changed regularly. And, by law, you must have the car pass inspection so that it is not a danger to you or others on the road. You comply.

Yet we, as a nation, continue to pump unhealthy, dangerous junk foods and drinks into our systems, knowing how we are harming ourselves. How and when did we decide that our cars are worth more than our own bodies?

But Americans love to blame heredity and medical conditions for obesity.

The reality is you're not lazy but you are tired. It's hard to imagine lacing up walking or running shoes for a two-mile walk when just finding the shoes is an exhausting exercise in of itself. As you read in Chapter Five about the "Fatty Liver," you understand that your lifestyle and choice of food/drink has begun a chain reaction leading to fatigue, bloat, and organs, such as the liver, no longer performing as they should. If this were your car, you would be appalled! You would make hasty arrangements to have the car looked at and fixed. As with the pregnancy.org dream team, attitude is everything. Once you begin to think of (and respect) yourself as a finely tuned machine, you can better appreciate how proper diet, exercise, sleep, and attitude can literally save your life.

3. Let's Get Real About Working Out

Question:
"I just found out I'm pregnant. But I have two problems. I'm overweight and I'm really out of shape. I want to start working out. I'm tired of always talking about it. I'm ready to start (I think!). What do I do?"

Answer:
First, pat yourself on the back. This is the starting point. Because you are a non-exerciser and are overweight, you need to see your doctor. I'm not passing the buck here but we need to be sure you do not have any medical conditions that should prevent you from working out. Once your doctor(s) gives permission to move forward, you should begin with low-impact cardio activities, such as walking or cycling. Start slowly and build up. Typically, my biggest concern with first-time exercisers is that they are gung-ho in the beginning, become very sore after the first couple of workouts and never exercise again.

A smart idea is always to contact a trainer, just to get started. But you can also get a buddy, significant other, family members, even a child to start a walking program with you. (See Part II: Chapter 9: The Controlled Workout).

Question:
"I'm finally pregnant. If I've never done anything before and start now, am I more likely to have a miscarriage?"

Answer:
A great question. Simply, no. But you must first get medical clearance to begin an exercise program. Once you get that green light, talk to a trainer or begin a walking program that is reasonable. Setting out on a 12-mile hike may not be the best of ideas for a previously sedentary person but a mile walk at a fairly challenging pace is the great beginning. From this, you can build the time and distance.

You will be pleased to note that studies show that women who begin an exercise program are actually less likely to have a miscarriage.

(Please re-read Chapter Four for safety guidelines)

When I talk to someone who isn't even pregnant about beginning an exercise program, I am tentative. Are they looking for immediate results? Do they not like to sweat? Personally, I always chuckle at that one! There are always the women in my classes who stop exercise as soon as they get too hot or begin to sweat too much because they don't want their make-up to run. But that's when the benefits are really kicking in!!! Argh!!

But when talking to a pregnant woman, my questions are more evasive. Are they working out in preparation of labor and delivery? Or to prevent weight gain?

It's time to get real about working out.

Both Dream Team candidates Beth and Cyndi worked out because they wanted to be sure they didn't gain too much weight during pregnancy. The key words: too much. They both understood that normal, healthy pregnancies require weight gain. But both women had hit on the most important reason for working out. Their babies. Beth and Cyndi both wanted to be good role models and have more energy for their children, in addition to having healthier, happier pregnancies.

You're not giving birth to footwear. Your number one reason for beginning a workout program and a lifestyle change should be for your baby. Your needs come second. Welcome to motherhood. Your health, weight, workouts, and attitude should be focused on your baby.

4. True Confessions of a Recovering Potato

The following sentiments are comments, notes, and pleas for help from recovering couch potatoes:

"I liked being pregnant. It was the one time in my life that I was allowed to eat whatever I wanted, sleep when I could without guilt, and be lazy. My husband was so happy we were pregnant, he would always tell me to take it easy. So I did.

I would get major cravings for sweet foods and things that were fried and salty. I told myself that this was okay since I was pregnant. And I told myself over and over again that whatever I put on, I would just take off later after the baby was born. So, I just kept on eating like I was pregnant with ten kids. I regret thinking that I could eat anything I wanted while I was pregnant. That's a big lie. You should tell people about that!"

"I kind of liked my big pregnant belly. People were always commenting about how good I looked or stuff like that. I started to believe what people were saying. But I know now that they were just saying that because I was so big. I gained so much weight and I never worked out. When it came time to have the baby, I was so tired and out of shape. I think that my labor was a lot longer and harder because I was so out of shape."

"Ha! I always read that when a mother breastfeeds that the weight would just "fall off." So I was thinking that if I put on too much weight it would be okay because it would just fall off after the baby was born. I gained over 50 pounds and all I did was eat junk food and candy. I made people at work go out and get me things all the time. Then when the baby was born and I was breastfeeding, my weight did not fall off. It just stayed there."

"I didn't work out because I thought it would be dangerous for the baby. That's what my mother-in-law told me. So I just watched t.v. and ate ALL THE TIME. I turned into a miserable whale but the worst was when I went to my husband's office party and there was a woman he worked with there who was pregnant. She looked so pretty. She looked really good and I asked her how far she was. She was one month more pregnant than I was! I couldn't believe it. She said that she went to aerobics three times a week and didn't eat any fast food. That was a real eye-opener for me."

"My mom always told me that your pregnancy was the one time in your life that you could do or eat anything you wanted so I took full advantage of that. She always talks about how she indulged herself when she was pregnant. She had four children. But she lived in a different time. She is Italian and for two of her pregnancies, she lived in Malta. No junk food, no cokes or kool-aid. Even when my parents came to America, she grew a big garden and almost everything she ate and cooked was organic. Of course, she gained like 20 pounds and then it melted away. I ate all the bad stuff and I gained nearly 60 pounds and 45 of it stayed with me after the baby was born. I don't think other countries have the same problems we do because they eat better and walk everywhere!"

It is true that American women are bombarded all day long with unhealthy choices. In Cedar Hill, Texas, (population 30,000), in less than one square acre there is a McDonalds, Schlotskies, Chicken Express, Popeye's Chicken, International House of Pancakes, Taco Bueno, Taco Bell, Whataburger, Sonic, … If that weren't enough, the medium sized city has an additional dozen or so restaurants in five-mile radius. This is just one city.

Radio, television, movie theaters, magazines and local newspapers all tout special "All You Can Eat!" deals and we haven't even discussed the giant push from soda manufacturers. It is overwhelming. And all the more reason to keep a journal, exercise, and stay focused on the needs of your baby.

But women from around the world all complain about the do-nothing-until-baby syndrome. No surprise, they are all shocked by how rebellious their body was after the baby was born. Except for the lucky few, weight does not "fall off."

5. Building Muscle

No matter how many times trainers, doctors, athletes, celebrities, and models all swear that building muscle does not automatically mean "bulk," some women hear the word "muscle" and shrink away. Fortunately, more and more women realize that lean, fit women have well-toned muscles and this is a good thing. But the word "muscle" doesn't always resonate well when talking about pregnancy.

Here's what you need to know about muscle and pregnancy: Most women's weight increases 15 to 25 percent while pregnant, putting a great deal of stress on her lower back, pelvis, hips, legs, and feet. Because of the enlarged abdomen, ligaments that once stabilized her hips, pelvis, and lower back are strained.

Your body responds in the most natural way. According to Dr. Clapp's extensive studies, both muscle mass and strength increase during this time in a woman's life, making her very receptive to a safe, low-impact workout. It is reasonable to conclude that your body wants and needs the stabilizing component of a stronger core – muscle. Despite what your mother told you, this is the time to get off the couch and begin working out!

Chapter Eight
Why Even Bother:
What's in It for You?

Pregnancy, labor, and delivery are hard work. Physical fitness helps not only the health and self-esteem of the mother, it helps the entire birthing process. Fit mothers have easier deliveries and healthier babies. They have labors that are one-third shorter, and they are much more likely to have normal vaginal births without complications. Exercising women are less likely to experience pre-eclampsia, also called pregnancy-induced hypertension, and gestational diabetes. And this is just the beginning.

I know it is hard to get started, particularly if you are tired. There is a reason I addressed anemia, fatty liver, diet, the ill-effects of caffeine, and weight in the previous pages. These issues alone can be draining you from any desire to exercise. But remember this: exercise is cyclical. You need energy to work out but once you work out, you will get more energy. If you can remember the end result promises more energy, perhaps this can motivate you to get started.

*Note: Energy stores are not created overnight! It will take you anywhere from two to four weeks to begin to see and feel the results of exercise.

1. The Benefits of Exercise for Labor and Delivery

Here's an attention grabber: Statistically speaking, you will have a faster, easier, healthier labor and delivery if your workout throughout your pregnancy. Women who remained active throughout their pregnancies have more than an 85 percent chance of having normal vaginal deliveries and labors that are one third shorter than non-exercisers. In short, exercising women deliver more quickly and easily with fewer complications than the non-exercising women. The use of forceps and the number of Cesarean sections were 300 percent greater among the non-exercising group.

This supports and is supported by a 1950 study by W.A. Pfeiffer which showed that of the 24 mothers who were Olympic athletes and/or world record holders, the majority had given birth quickly and easily. Their deliveries were shorter and they, upon return to their athletic competitions, were stronger athletes. Pfeiffer believed that the hormones activated by pregnancy might account for the easier deliveries and improvement in athletic performances.

2. The Beneficial Baby

Question:
"I've read that babies are better off or healthier if their moms work out when they are pregnant. Is this true?"

Answer:
You bet. Across the board, moms-to-be report that the more they worked out while pregnant the more energetic and healthier they felt but there were direct benefits for the baby as well.

Babies of exercising moms are reportedly leaner, more intelligent and curious. They have better verbal, cognitive and analytical skills. To this, I have often laughed that my daughter Katie, the bobsled baby, is the walking poster child to support why moms should exercise while pregnant. A lean machine, she was saying "photosythisis" when she was five years old.

Babies of exercising mothers also have half as many instances of abnormal heart rate and in utero bowel movements (both a sign of stress) as did the babies of sedentary moms.

As Katie was part of Dr. Clapp's extensive research, the best news is that babies of mothers who exercise continue to have less body fat than those babies of the non-exercising group.

Question:
"I feel guilty. I am talking so much about being healthy for this pregnancy but I didn't do that for my last one. I don't want my 2-year-old to think he's less important than this pregnancy!"

Answer:
Quite the opposite. He's not too young to understand that mommy is exercising to get healthy for the entire family. And, in fact, as you exercise more, you will find that you are more patient with your toddler. You will feel more relaxed, more calm, and happy. Thus, you are already being a better mom to your little one.

Invite him to workout with you. Together, you can take walks. Invest in a jogger stroller – a great workout to push the combined weight of your son and the stroller. Give him soup cans and let him "flex" and "work the biceps" with you. Pop in a yoga video and stretch together. It's a great way to bond with your toddler.

3. Baby Blues

Low self-esteem can attack when you least expect it. Despite the "glow" of your pregnancy, the now-rounding belly can represent other things besides life. Many women become depressed, scared, or anxious.

Exercise is an important health factor in a pregnant woman's self-esteem. Women who exercise during pregnancy have more energy and more positive body images than women who don't. They report more positive attitudes about their hips, facial complexion, energy level, body build, and health than sedentary women. They also have more positive feelings about their sex lives, while sedentary women report significantly more negative feelings about sexual activities. And because a woman who works out tends to be in tune with her body, she is less likely to become depressed.

It is important to note that the mood of the mother can affect the fetus. Research at the University of Miami School of Medicine found that 10 percent of women depressed during pregnancy transmitted this depression to their babies (who grew from depressed infants to depressed toddlers, until the conditions were chronic).

This said, however, it is important that you know everyone is different. Pregnancy is not a guaranteed state of bliss. Approximately 70 percent of women who are pregnant or recently had a baby feel some form of depression that includes weepiness, anxiety, and unexplained sadness. Don't be embarrassed. Talk to your physician about your feelings and give yourself a break.

It is important that you understand this may not simply be a matter of "sucking it up." Hormonal influxes are real. Deep emotion, depression, anxiety, and stress are so real, in fact, they can cause harmful medical problems. Do not delay in speaking to a professional about your feelings.

4. Muscle Memory

Another reason to work out is because of the recovery after your baby is born. When your body is acclimated to specific movements and exercises, it will happily accept – okay, maybe not always happily – a harder, more intense workout later on down the road. By working out while you are pregnant, you are laying excellent groundwork for later training days...

Recently, I told a client we were going to start running two miles. She looked at me as though I was speaking Swahili. I knew three things about her when I suggested this. One, she was out of shape but strong. Two, we would be walking more than we would be running – but it's a start. And three, she has muscle memory.

"Muscle memory?" she quipped. "I don't remember having any muscle!"

She's 50 pounds overweight with a bad knee and ankle and has tried a variety of diets. She's tried low-carb, no carb, low-calories, no sugar, all veggies, 3-a-day apples, and more. Nothing has worked and her weight and joints continue to plague her. Somewhere along the way, she gave up on the idea of burning calories. It's easy to do when your knee screams and your ankle groans each time you run. And it's easy to do when you're embarrassed about the idea of working out.

"I kept thinking that if I could be a certain weight or size," she said, "then it wouldn't be so bad to work out. But I just didn't want anyone to see me at the weight I was before working out."

Then, she came to realize that a diet is just a band-aid. Working out, sweating, burning calories, pumping the heart, and getting the blood flowing is the true answer to permanent weight loss. Still, she had been suspicious. What is muscle memory and how in the world was it going to help her?

Muscle memory is a term many athletes use when talking about coming back from a pregnancy. But the idea isn't new, nor is it limited to elite athletes. During the 1960s and 70s, the Russians held the philosophy that female athletes once having had a baby, came back stronger because they endured childbirth. The Russians believed that becoming a mother made athletes more dedicated and responsible about training time, but also gave them better endurance and power. The United States did not adopt this philosophy until the late 1980s but is was not until the mid-1990s that the idea of muscle memory applied to everyday moms.

Your body remembers and retains the 'how-to' information on running, leaping, swinging, swimming, biking, reaching, and jumping. While you may get tired, and your leaps may not be quite the leaps they once were, your body knows what to do and will regain the form you once had with practice. Recovery is made much easier.

According to Dr. Clapp, the recovery rate of women who exercised during pregnancy and "get their lives back in order," is about fifty percent faster than the women who did not exercise.

5. Better Moms, Better Children

The benefits of motherhood mixed with sports are limitless. Throughout this chapter, you read how exercise will help you and your baby during and after pregnancy. But the benefits go beyond infant and toddler years. It's inevitable that our children learn from our examples. This is your time to make life changes. The way you eat and exercise will spill over into your child's lifestyle.

Your children will also learn to be more disciplined and more focused, as they watch their moms (and their dads), maintain commitment to their activity of choice – whether it's recreational or professional. It is important to show our children that we can do anything we set our minds to – that determination is half the battle, and perseverance is the other half. (And this attitude is extremely important when it comes time to breastfeed!)

Women who worked out during pregnancy have given their children one of the best tools for starting out in life: lower body fat. During the first year of life the number of fat cells increases fairly rapidly. It is estimated that the fat cells are three times greater at one year than at birth, and that the last three months of pregnancy are the critical periods for the baby.

Physically, there are three critical periods in the young human's life that are really up to the mothers. The first is during the mother's pregnancy, during the last trimester. What she eats and how she exercises greatly affect the fat cells in the baby. The second is during the baby's first years of life. What the baby is fed is crucial. The third period for the child is puberty.

While taking care of ourselves, we have ultimately taken care of our babies, both the born and unborn. Our healthy lifestyles have set the groundwork for generations to come.

6. Team Baby

Think of journaling as "me" time. Take just a few moments to record your daily meals and snacks, how you slept, and where/how you worked out. This daily routine helps you better understand your body, your moods, your workouts, and potential problems (e.g the onset of a cold).

Be sure to show your journal to everyone on Team Baby. Show your doctor, OB/GYN, trainer, nutritionist, workout buddy, even family. As other people see your goals and progress, you will feel empowered and garner more support.

Part II: Working Out or Finding Your Sport While Pregnant

Chapter 9:
The Controlled Workout

What is a controlled workout? For our purposes, a controlled workout is one that can minimize unpreventable accidents, such as dog bites, car accidents, or black ice. When you cycle indoors we can control the room temperature, opportunities to check your inner core temperature, guarantee workout buddies (or certainly people nearby to assist you should you need any help) and, outside of the freak accident of a ceiling fan falling on you, know that you are out of harms way. Even as I write this, my daughter and I are recovering from a near miss on the road. While I ran, my daughter rode her bicycle alongside of me, keeping me company with her endless stories. I'd noticed an oncoming car, a might too close to our side of the road and quickly instructed Katie to get on the very edge of the road. As the car loomed, I saw a very young driver behind the wheel, apparently reaching for some lost items. With no recourse, I lunge forward, shoving Katie from her bike and the two of us toppled into a ditch.

A teenage girl, most likely searching for her cell phone, a CD, or make-up, was leaned over to the right of her car and NEVER saw us. After that harrowing episode, she still never stopped, slowed, or looked back.

Man!!

The point is, when you exercise outdoors there are a number of potential dangers. From dogs and cars to heat exhaustion and poor weather conditions, this is not the time in your life to have to run for cover or flag down cars for help.

Question:

"My wife is four months pregnant and I'm worried about her getting hurt while exercising. I've heard people say that when women get pregnant, they get clumsy and can get hurt. She's not clumsy now but should I be concerned about her riding bikes, which she loves to do?"

Answer:

This is a great question. Scientifically, the answer is … well, mixed. Extensive studies have shown that women's equilibriums do tend to be off (the new shift in weights tends to make women clumsier), and their ligaments and pelvic joints are stretching and loosening in preparation for delivery (which makes them more susceptible to accidental injuries like sprained ankles and overuse injuries like tendonitis).

However, women who work out tend to use more caution and pay more attention to their bodies and how they respond to exercise, thus reducing the instances of injury.

You can certainly understand why fitness experts prefer stationary bikes over riding outdoors or treadmills over running the streets in your neighborhood.

1. The Machines: Stairmaster, Elliptical, Treadmill, and Cycling

Question:
"When I use the Stairmaster, I stay on it until I'm dripping with sweat. Now that I'm pregnant, I want to know if I can still keep doing that?"

Answer:
Can you continue to use the Stairmaster? You bet. But we'll need to make a few changes. Once you've been given permission from your doctor to continue, you must be willing to make a few mild adjustments. The good news is you are obviously acclimated to this activity and can easily handle the workload while pregnant. Because the Stairmaster and elliptical, to name a few, are very low-impact, I am not concerned about any pounding on your joints as you progress in your pregnancy. But I am concerned about heat.

It is important that if you are on the Stairmaster for a significant amount of time that you stop to check your inner core temperature to be sure you are in the safety zone. To remind you, you do not want to exceed 101 degree F.

Let's say you use the Stairmaster for 20 minutes at a moderate pace – and you just happen to sweat a lot. You can continue this current program if 1) you are properly hydrated and have water with you, 2) have permission from your doctor to continue, and 3) feel strong and healthy while you are doing this. As you progress in your pregnancy, you may naturally decide to drop back on time and/or intensity.

But if you are doing30+ minutes at a harder pace, you will need to check your inner core temperature the first 15 to 20 minutes and every ten minutes after that. We need to be sure that you do not have a temperature spike or unwittingly fatigue yourself. Making yourself stop to check your inner core temperature is a safety measure you should be willing to make for your baby!

I've had women complain that once they step off the Stairmaster, they lose the equipment because the gym is so pack. Just because you might lose your turn, do not forgo checking your inner core temperature!

The body of a pregnant woman is ever evolving, ever-changing. Ligaments and pelvic joints are stretching and loosening in preparation for delivery. Besides the topic of inner core temperature, the previous statement is probably my second more favorite because pregnant women (and their trainers) tend to forget the amazing and traumatic things that occur while a woman is pregnant. For this reason, I am a fan of the low-impact machines.

Again, they allow you to be in a temperature controlled room with bathrooms, water fountains, and people. As for the machines, they are easier on the joints and ligaments.

How to Use the Machines

- Do not lean or hang on Stairmasters, treadmills, or ellipticals. If you must lean forward, you are losing proper form. This puts a strain on your body and develops poor work habits. If you must, bring down the level of intensity until you can recover proper form.
- Keep your head up, back straight.
- When/if using the treadmill, be very cautious after third trimester. Perhaps you should move to the stationary bike, elliptical or stairmaster! The moving belt on the treadmill could be a hazard if you misstep.

Question:
"I've never used any of the machines in the gym before. My husband and I just joined a gym and now I'm pregnant. Can I even use anything? I'm afraid to try."

Answer:
Don't be! This is a great time to utilize all that the gym offers. You need to:
1. Get permission from your doctor
2. Talk to the gym manager – explain that you've never really worked out before and that you are pregnant.
3. Acclimate yourself to the equipment. If you choose, for example, the elliptical, have a couple of trial runs on the elliptical (warm-ups of 5 to 10 minutes) before you call this your "cardio" workout. Then try the treadmill, stationary bikes, and Stairmaster. Don't get stuck on just one kind of machine.

Once you get comfortable, choose your cardio workout of choice. Now, here's where it is critical for you to work with a trainer and begin a safe program for cardio.

1. Don't look around at other people, pedaling or running 80 miles per hour and thinking you have to keep up. Pick your own pace, however pokey, and let that be your starting point.

2. Don't be a slacker! I always have clients who have deluded themselves into thinking because they are physically moving that they are working out. You want to reach a point where you are heating up, you can feel your body having to work to sustain a certain speed or level. If you are merrily chatting to your neighbor about a movie you saw last night you're not working that hard. Remember the talk test? You want to be able to talk but it should be slightly challenging.
3. Working with your trainer, determine either a time or distance you will put in on the machine. 10 minutes. 15 minute. 20 minutes. One mile. Three miles. Half a mile. With a trainer nearby, you can determine your anaerobic threshold and what is reasonable for you to begin with.

This is your starting point. Over the course of your pregnancy, you may be surprised by what happens. As a novice to the machines, you may actually increase your times and distances, even while pregnant!! Because you are new to all this, you will be ever building in your quest for better cardio.

Question:
"I've read where you tell people to check their inner core temperature after about 15 minutes on the treadmill and then every ten minutes after that but you tell other people to check themselves every 20 minutes. What is the difference?"

Answer:
Well, it's good to see you're paying attention! Yes, I do recommend that people new to exercise check their inner core temperature after about fifteen minutes of exercise to be sure they have not exceeded 101 degree F.

Because they are new to exercise and do not know what to expect from their bodies or reaction to exercise, I urge them to check their temperatures again every ten minutes for the remainder of their exercise routine. Why? Because they could very well have a spike or sudden rise in their body temperature without even knowing it.

I also urge women to keep a fitness journal. Each time you check your inner core temperature, write it down. Over time, you can see (and compare) your inner core temperature in correlation to specific exercises and times/distances.

For the more seasoned runners, every 20 minutes is the most realistic expectation for them to stop and check their temperature.

Question:
"I did what you said and started running on the treadmill instead of outside. It seems a lot easier and I was able to run 1 mile straight on the treadmill. It felt easier than outside and I was definitely able to go further. I've never run 1 mile straight before!! Why is that?"

Answer:

That's fantastic! Feels great, doesn't it? Obviously, there are a great many hills and declines/inclines outside but even the more subtle grooves in the road, the slight curve, dips, and turns make the run a harder one. The treadmill offers a straight, smooth run, making it easier to run that mile.

If you were training for a 5k, 10k or half-marathon, I would urge you to hit the road. Figuratively speaking. You would need those inclines to build muscle and stamina. But this is a great workout for you while pregnant. While working on the treadmill, you can slowly begin working on your times and distances.

*Remember! Your body is always changing. Using the treadmill is a great alternative to running outside. But as you get bigger and feel less sure-footed, I would urge you to use the elliptical or Stairmaster where you are less likely to stumble or catch a foot half-off the belt on the treadmill.

The rule of thumb still exists with the exercise equipment. You may continue doing whatever you were doing before you got pregnant. As long as you have your doctor's permission, you can still do those 20-, 30-, and 40-minute workouts on the machines, following these rules:

- Stop to check your inner core temperature
- Record those temperatures in your journal
- Stay hydrated
- Use common sense. Listen to your body.
- Don't worry what your training buddies or neighbors are doing
- Don't worry about slowing down. Muscle memory will be your best friend later on.

If you are new to training on cardio machines:

- Start slowly, working with a trainer or training buddy
- Pick a reasonable pace that both challenges you but does not make you so breathless you are unable to speak
- Pick a reasonable distance or time as you begin
- Record your efforts in a journal
- Each week try to add a little time or distance. How much? Try adding 100 extra steps from your last effort.
- Stop to check your inner core temperature
- Stay hydrated

- Stop if you experience any discomfort and talk to your trainer about these feelings. He or she will help you determine what is normal exercise-induced fatigue and what is out of the norm
- Do not get into a contest. Move at your own pace and TRULY enjoy this time for yourself!

Love Thy Treadmill

The biggest myth concerning the treadmill is that it is boring. It can only be boring if the routine is boring. The reality is, the treadmill is one of the best pieces of equipment you can use to keep your training routine fresh and challenging. While pregnant, it is a sure way to control your environment. It really is all in the way you use it!

While training for her tough-girl role in "G.I. Jane," Demi Moore was on the treadmill from one to two hours a day. While her results were amazing, her routine was boring. Most of us don't have millions of dollars as incentive to stick with such a routine and not stray. But there are other ways to love the treadmill and the results it will ultimately bring.

Whether you are an Olympian or 9-5-desk jockey, you must ask yourself what your goals are. Before you answer, remember that you are pregnant. You are not doing this for a flat stomach or killer thighs. What you should be looking for is better endurance, a stronger frame and metabolism. With your doctor's permission, you can set up walking or jogging programs for the treadmill. Hit the treadmill with the idea that you are building to a timed goal. Three times a week, set your pace for a five-minute warm-up.

If you are new to the exercise game, it's recommended that you work with a trainer to determine what a good distance and time should be for you. I cannot emphasis enough that this is **not** the time to "suck it up" and "be tough." I want you to enjoy a walking (or jogging) routine. I want you to safely and slowly build a strong cardio routine.

If you can only walk ten minutes, build on this. As mentioned previously, simply begin adding 100 additional steps, then start looking at your distances. You will be amazed how quickly your body will adapt and be willing to take on more.

However, if you are more hardcore than this, try this on for size:

*remember that this particular routine is for more of an elite athlete. The numbers should be adjusted to your fitness level. You can also create a similar routine with walking:

Sample routine:

    5 minutes – warm up
    2 minutes – 3.0 MPH jog
    2 minutes – 3.4 MPH jog
    30 seconds -- 4.0 MPH jog/sprint
    2 minutes – 3.2 MPH recovery jog
    2 minutes – 3.4 MPH jog
    1 minute -- 4.5 MPH sprint
    2 minutes – 3.4 MPH recovery jog (stay longer if needed)
        *If needed, reduce speed but increase incline so that you are
         walking/hiking at a hard angle
    2 minutes – 4.3 MPH jog
    1 minute -- 4.5 MPH Sprint
    2 minutes – 2.3 MPH recovery
    7 minutes – 3.5 MPH jog

    *hold a steady jog for next seven to 10 minutes
    1 minute – 4.5 MPH sprint
    2 minute – 2.5 MPH recovery
    1 minute – 3.0 MPH jog
    1 minute - 3.7 MPH sprint
    2 minutes – 3.0 MPH recovery
    1 minute – 3.5 MPH jog
    2 minutes –3.0 MPH jog
    1 minute -- 4.3 MPH sprint
    2 minutes – 3.5 MPH jog
    1 minute -- 4.5 MPH sprint
    2 minutes – 2.5 recovery
    30 seconds – 2.0 walk it off …
                    = 45 minutes

*Again, this is an example for a seasoned runner. I even urge that the elite runner move to the stationary bike, elliptical or Stairmaster into the third trimester for safety reasons. It is easy to misstep as your middle grows! Be careful.

2. The Traditional 50-minute Cardio Class

Question:
"I have just found out that I am pregnant and was wondering if I would be able to continue kickboxing. My husband and I have gone around and around about

whether it is safe for me to continue. He says no. What do you think? Will all that punching and kicking hurt me or the baby?"

Answer:

Of course, you must first speak to your doctor to be sure there are no medical problems that might prevent you from working out or being a high risk pregnancy. But if he or she gives you the green light to exercise AND you are already used to the activity of kickboxing, there is no reason to quit! Kickboxing is truly one of the best forms of exercise. Not only does it tone and define muscle but it develops better balance, builds self-esteem, and is the "thinking persons" form of exercise. That is, you are less likely to become bored with a good kickboxing instructor.

That said, let's go over some ground rules. Even in the beginning of your pregnancy, I would urge you to hold back on your punches and kicks on the heavy bags. You can and should continue to punch and kick but not nearly with the same ferocity you did before. Why? Two reasons: I want you to get into the habit of pulling back. Right now you are very strong. There is no question about that. But as you move along in your pregnancy, your joints will loosen and your ligaments will soften. As they do, if you are still pounding and kicking away on the heavy bags, this could cause hip, groin, leg, or upper body injuries. Now is the time to be working on form rather than power.

By the second trimester, I really don't allow my pregnant women to punch and kick at 100 percent. Fifty percent is all you need. You're still moving around the bag, learning to keep your guards up, working the jabs, and working the feet. You do not need the jarring that occurs when hitting the bag.

By your third trimester, I like for you to tap/touch the bag. While touching, you can absolutely get a hard workout, working speed. I conduct many classes where the rule is "touch only!" so that people can work on proper form, speed and balance rather than brute strength. Any caveman can charge a bag and whale on it. But do you have finesse? Can you string four or five strikes and counters together?

- You must stop to check your inner core temperature during class.
- You must tell your instructor that you are pregnant.
- You must tell a few people in your class that you are pregnant. Because your instructor is dealing with multiple students and tasks, s/he can't always look after you. Allow others to know and give their friendly/concerned observations that you appear to be flushed or red-faced with an open heart. This is for the good of both you and baby.
- Do not get into a contest of "being tough."
- Enjoy yourself and take this time to develop your skills rather than power!

Not all instructors are created equal!

Unless your group instructor took an intense interest in obstetrics, the chances are, he or she is limited in knowledge regarding pregnancy and training. Most group certifications merely touch on the subject of exercise and pregnancy. They learn about the benefits of exercise to the woman and fetus and how to protect the lower back. Certified instructors are shown the ACOG's guidelines, the suggested weight gain for pregnant women, and given a description of Kegel exercises.

A big focus is on oxygen, explaining, "Pregnant women ventilate 50% more air per minute than non-pregnant women. This occurs through a 40% - 50% increase in tidal volume, or the amount of air in each breath. Although many pregnant women feel it is difficult to get a deep breath, maximum breathing capacity is actually maintained or increased over pre-pregnancy values. Respiratory rate does not change significantly. As the baby grows, the uterus pushes the diaphragm farther up into the chest cavity. The pregnant woman has to use more oxygen during inspiration as the diaphragm contracts to push the uterus downward. This increase in the oxygen is available to the working muscles." (ACE, 253.)

Most certified instructors know the dangers of overheating but are not savvy to how to determine that inner core temperature.

Be aware that while you may have an incredibly fun, energetic, and aerobically fit instructor who knows goo-boos about static strength, trunk flexors, or the law of acceleration, s/he may not be completely comfortable on the subject of mommas-in-training.

Your best trainer, your best friend, and your very best guide is common sense.

Question:
"I'm pregnant but I don't want to have to give up my step-aerobics! I think I would miss my friends in that class as much as I would the exercise. Do I have to stop because of all the bouncing?"

Answer:
Stop the class? No way. Stop the bouncing? Well …

I am so pleased to hear you are so thrilled with your class, I would not dream of stopping that! Half the battle for most exercisers is getting excited about an activity. And as your pregnancy continues – thus making you more and more tired – you will really want that class and those friends to cheer you on.

But we have a few "buts" to iron out. Uh.. well, you know what I mean.

Of course, you need to get permission to continue with this class from your doctor. You also need to let your instructor and aerobic buddies know that you are pregnant and be sure to clue them into the "inner core temperature" and "stay hydrated" rules.

As your pregnancy progresses, you may want/need to trade in your 4 or 5-pound hand weights for lighters ones and, you will want to lose the step.

By minimizing the bouncing, you are doing your body a favor down the road. It is easy to believe that you "can handle" the bouncing but with each bounce, you are pulling or stressing the abdominal ligaments – ligaments, by the way, that are already being stretched throughout your pregnancy.

You know that catchy little diddy … "Ohhh, the broad ligaments are connected to the round ligaments and the round ligaments are connected to the …"

Okay, forget the song but know that truly, everything is connected.

Round ligaments can be irritated by extreme stretching overhead, jogging, jumping (i.e. bouncing), or rapid twisting movements. As the round ligaments connects to both sides of the uterus fundus (where it may feel all the action of baby is), women will often feel the strain of what these ligaments have been through toward the end of the pregnancy. You want to BUILD a strong body, not tear down while pregnant.

Your largest ligament supporting the ovaries, uterus, and vagina is the broad ligament. As we will discuss later, this is a great reason to perform slow, relaxing stretches and pelvic tilts to give relieve and gently build muscle. The idea here is to be sure that you've not stretched or pulled ligaments beyond repair and that your post-pregnancy recovery is fast and painless.

Question:
"I find myself at a crossroad. I just found out that I am expecting my second child. I have been in Kung Fu for several years now and have been in training for my black sash test. Although I was ecstatic when I found out I was pregnant, my heart sank with the thought of having to cut back on my physical workouts. I spoke to my instructor and I could test with no sparring. This would put me at about 13 to 14 weeks. Some of my friends think I am crazy to risk it, but for me it's a goal that I have been waiting to attain for so long. Of course, I dread the thought of causing complications with my pregnancy and the fetus. I have heard stories of female athletes, going to the Olympics at four months. I am 35 years old now. I'm already in a higher risk bracket. I guess my question is obvious. Is it possible to continue training and actually take my black sash test when I am 13 to 14 months pregnant?

Answer:

The great news here is that there are many Olympic athletes, in their 30s, who trained while pregnant. In fact, I was a 34 years old, I tested for my second black belt in tae kwon do.

But there are some things you must consider . . .

Throughout my training, I made sure I drank plenty of fluids and checked my inner core temperature. This is easy to do and does not (really) impede your training times. It is important because your baby is 1 degree Celcius hotter than you and has no sweating mechanism. You want to be sure you do not exceed 101 degrees F while working out. My body was acclimated to what I was doing so it wasn't as though I was jumping into a new and strenuous program. You have been doing this a long time and are well adjusted to the demands of your sport.

I was sure never to reach a high anaerobic level – high heart rate – for more than 10 seconds. As long as you heart rate is not elevated beyond a reasonable rate for a long period of time, you are in the safe zone. I would certainly not advise this exercise for someone new to the sport but you've been waived of any sparring (excellent! We don't want you sparring!) and can continue with form rather than physical contact.

Of course, you have to have medical permission. We need to be sure that there is not a medical history that could cause problems for you/baby. But if you can keep your inner core temperature in check and have medical permission, you should be able to realize this goal. Good luck.

Question:

"I do kickboxing and have done so off and on for approximately 9 years. I stopped during my first pregnancy which resulted in a caesarean four years ago. I am now 12 weeks pregnant and continue to kickbox on a one to one basis at a lower intensity. My concern is as I get into my pregnancy and continue to engage in kickboxing how will it impinge on my existing c-section and what precautions I would need to take."

Answer

Great question! Because you had a c-section, you want to watch irritating the scar tissue. The benefits of kickboxing are plentiful in terms of preparing for labor & delivery. You will have better endurance, stamina, upper and lower body strength to push/grip. During the kickbox pregnancy, however, you want to be sure you don't over-stretch, strain your joints or dehydrate. Let's break it down: Because you've kickboxed for so many years, you already know that you will burn more calories in 45 minutes of kickbox than almost any other exercise. This also means your inner core temperature will spike. Please check out our information on inner core temperature and how you can continuously check it throughout your workouts. Remember that your baby has no sweating mechanism and is 1 degree Celsius hotter than your own inner core temp. This is important information because you need to know that by overheating, you are spiking the baby's temperature. You can continue to train safely and happily -- but watch your temperature. Check out our information on inner core temp.

In kickbox, as with any exercise class, there seems to be some silent rule that you can't leave the class. Do not feel trapped by your classmates. Periodically stop, walk to the locker rooms or water fountain and get a drink. By doing so, you are staying hydrated but are also helping your body regulate heat.

You also need to be aware of your previous cesarean (or c-section) scars. By working quick twitch fibers -- the rapid succession of kicking -- you are really working lower abdominal muscles. Add to this, any of the deep reaching/stretching you may be doing while punching the bag or hitting a small target pad. In these cases, there really is such a thing as too much of a good thing. If/when you are asked to do higher repetitions of kicks -- anything over 12 -- keep your kicks at the number twelve and lower the kicks slightly. This will help decrease the kind of friction your muscles/scar tissue will incur while working out.

When you punch, hook, upper cut, lunge, or side-to-side squat, minimize the intensity. You may certainly go through the motions but make them precise, fluid, and concentrate more on form rather than power. When it comes to front kicks, hook and round kicks, keep the numbers slightly lower and use this time to really concentrate on form and balance.

I always tell my pregnant clients -- don't look at this as a time when you "can't keep up with the class" or "have to slow down." Look at this as a time of real development. Most kickboxers do not get proper technique because the music is jamming and the class is rocking and everyone is moving rapidly and aggressively -- translation: sloppy form. And sloppy form means higher chance of injury, less muscular workout, less chance of learning the higher form of self-defense.

Use this as a time to look at your form, your feet, foot placement. For example, the standard sidekick. In pictures of kickboxers around the nation always shows a woman doing her best "hi-ya!" impression as she does a side kick. Look at her toes. They are almost always pointing up toward the ceiling and her rear end is sticking out as she is bent forward.

WRONG!!!!!!

A good, solid sidekick has you standing almost erect, shoulders back, head up and when you kick, the foot is parallel to the floor -- toes down and pulled back toward your own body. The idea here is that should you ever have to really kick someone, you are pulling your toes back so that they won't break against the target. A kick with the toes are up toward the ceiling is a front kick.

You get the idea.

If your instructor does not teach proper form -- and don't worry -- most do not because they have a background in aerobics, not martial arts, trot on over to your local book store and check out some martial arts -- very basic -- to learn proper form.

Finally, and we've already touched on this somewhat, your joints and ligaments are loosening/softening during your pregnancy. This is another reason I would like to see you focus on form rather than intensity and brute strength. To prevent injury, simply enjoy the art of kickbox, focus on form and have a great time.

Question:

"My husband and I are trying to conceive and I jog regularly. But I miss my martial arts class. I stopped but hoped to start up again. Still, I wonder how the training will affect conception. I feel almost silly asking but if an egg gets fertilized and attaches itself to the uterine wall, can body contact during training (such as kicks to the stomach during sparring) cause it to detach? Or affect it another way?"

Answer:

You can practice martial arts without sparring. Sparring (fighting) is but just one aspect of martial arts.

As you learn forms, balance, and patterns, you will also develop muscle, stamina, and friendships. As you are trying to conceive, let me assure you that it is extremely unlikely that such a kick would "detach" anything. It's not a silly question and you are wise to look to the future. You can ensure your own safety by talking to the instructor. Explain that while you want to learn martial arts, you are also hoping to conceive and do not wish to have any contact/fighting with other students. A good instructor will not only understand this but will readily take on the challenge of focusing on the true art-form of martial arts.

Question:

"I've been taking a cardio bootcamp class for over two years and love it! But with all the sit-ups, squats, jumps, and running around, I worry that it is too much. I am four weeks pregnant and need to know if this is safe to continue."

Answer:

These kind of intense classes can really spike your inner core temperature without you ever realizing how hot you actually are. Because you do so much kicking -- using the largest muscles in your body (your legs) -- thereby requiring a great deal of oxygen -- your internal temperature can jump before you even begin to sweat or realize how hard you've been working.

First, you need to talk to your doctor. Do not simply mention, "Oh, I also take a cardio bootcamp class ..." Be sure to lay out exactly what it is you do. Because I do know your medical history or physical condition, it's important that you clue in your doctors as to what you are doing. However, let's assume that your physician has talked to you, reviewed your medical history and knows what you are doing in the bootcamp class, and gives you permission to continue. With this green light, there are things you should do to continue the safety of you/your baby.

1) Drink plenty of fluids -- water. I know, I know... you hear this all the time. But most American women are dehydrated and don't even know it. It is important -- more so than ever -- that you stay hydrated. Staying hydrated will reduce morning sickness, leg cramps, and help cool your body.

It is a great idea to simply walk off, get some water, catch your breath and allow your body a few minutes to recover when needed.

2) Tell your instructor that you are pregnant. He or she should keep an eye on you, remind you to get water, and modify some of the routines/exercises as you grow. But because your instructor cannot always watch you, be sure to tell your fellow classmates as well.

3) Watch your inner core temperature. This is the single most important thing you can do. What is inner core temperature?? First, let me say this... kickboxing and cardio bootcamp classes are some of the most intense, calorie-burning exercises you can do. As a result, your body heat soars. Yes, I know you feel the sweat but often times, it is your inner core temperature that can spike without

Your baby is 1 degree Celsius hotter than your own temperature. But, baby has no sweating mechanism to cool his or her little self down. Therefore, as you get hotter and hotter, so does the baby. As a general rule of safety, you should not allow your body temperature to exceed 101 degree F.

Thus, the question: So, how do I check to make sure I don't exceed 101 degree F?

Answer: (brace yourself -- it's icky) Rectal thermometer.

You can get it in any pharmacy. Carry it with you in a little cute bag. As you are 15-20 minutes into the intense training, dash off to the bathroom and check your temp. It's that simple. I know, I know.. it's icky but this will give you great peace of mind, will make your instructor happy, and, most importantly, will let you know that your baby is in the safety zone. Halfway through the class, check your temperature again.

I've been asked, "Yeah, but can't I just tell if I'm really hot?" No. You cannot judge your inner core temperature by how much you are or aren't sweating. It doesn't work that way and you shouldn't want to guess.

I also suggest keeping an exercise/diet journal while you are pregnant. Write down inner core temps along with whatever the exercise routine was to help you gauge what makes your inner core temperature rise... you will begin to get a better feel for what's safe and what's just too much as you exercise and as the baby grows.

4) Watch your heart rate. Gone are the days that we tell women they can't allow their heart rate to go over 140 beats per minute. For women who are already in great shape and work out regularly, they can go beyond 140 beats per minute, however, there are a few guidelines here.

As I mentioned: You must be in good shape, a regular exercise buff and be acclimated to the exercise routine. Now, for example, is not the time to try out strong yoga. Stick with what your body knows. And, however conditioned you are, do not allow your heart rate to rise and stay there. You can allow your heart rate to rise for about 20-30 seconds, then you must come back down again.

You will see a lot of elite pregnant athletes talk about "sprint" training. The sprint is short-lived, allowing them to immediately look to recovery. In this case, recovery means catching your breath. Once your heart rate is high, bring it back down, walk off and get a drink of water!

5) Don't compete! I see this a lot. Pregnant women are animals! They love the exercise and love showing how strong they are. Yes, you are really strong while pregnant. But, this can unwittingly become a problem as competitive moms-to-be are determined to show they can hang with the class. Don't get caught up in this. Drink your water and check your inner core temp. That's your main priority.

Now, let's talk about sit ups and squats.

Right now, I am assuming that you are acclimated to this exercise regimen and, again, that you have been given permission from your doctor. At four weeks, you can continue your sit ups. It's advised that in the second trimester, moms begin doing side sit ups. This takes pressure away from the spine but allows you to continue working your core. Again, please talk to your instructor about this. I want to be sure that you are not tugging or jerking while you do the sit ups. [See Proper Sit-Up Form in Part III].

Squats. I don't recommend jump squats, however you can get a fantastic workout from standing squats with low weights. Even then, it is crucial that you speak to your doctor and work with a trainer. Improper form or too heavy of a weight could cause problems. Have your instructor show you the proper form while squatting. It is imperative that you own a good form as your body is going to be changing quite a bit. We want to be sure that you protect your lower back.

Finally, as you grow, your body joints will loosen. This is natures' way of preparing you for childbirth. For this reason, I do not like to see women punching or kicking HARD on a bag. It's time to scale back on the intensity. The impact on your body from punching/kicking can be too much.

Question:
"My husband I are hoping to conceive and I have some questions about my current workout and continuing it through pregnancy. I am 5ft 1.5 in, 100 lbs, very active and have very good nutrition (local organic meats, huge vegetable garden, etc) Here is my current workout:
- *M, F: NordicTrack (30-50 min) at varied intensities or cycling on a rail trail @ 15 mph for an hour. A 30-40 min Pilates video, Ana Caban, Hilary Burnett or Stott -- Intermediate; Tai Chi 10-15 min; some jumping/plyometric type exercises 10 min*
- *W: 30min-1.5 hr walk, lots of stretching*
- *T, R: 40-50 min Lift weights (pulleys and dumb-bells, sometimes plate machines) a good mix of functional (lunges with 30 lbs, woodchops and lawn-mower pulls, etc) and stuff like bicep curls, deltoid raises, etc. Swim laps 20-30 min. Stretch*
- *Weekend: Ski, Nordic Ski, road biking, Hike, Garden, kayak, depending on the weather.*

I would like to continue with the assumption that if we get pregnant, sometimes I might be too tired. What are your recommendations? I'd also like some recommendations for Pilates for pregnancy videos that don't assume that the viewer has no fitness!"

Answer:

You are in great shape and are committed to a solid workout routine. That's excellent. What you are doing now will greatly benefit your health and that of your baby-to-be. But some things will have to change after you've become pregnant. First, let's put your mind at ease.

The good news is, your workouts -- while intense -- are low impact. Excellent! Because you are already conditioned to a strong workout routine, you need not worry.

I must tell you that you need to get your physicians permission. Because I do not know your medical history/background, medications you may be taking, prior injuries... I must insist that you get permission from your personal doctor. Be sure to show him or her your workout routine. Having said this (and assuming that you are given a good health report), there is nothing here to indicate you need to stop. Let's break it all apart.

Nordic track. Great workout, low impact, high intensity. Again, you are conditioned for this so I don't have to worry about you trying something new or straining muscles. But you must watch your inner core temperature. Please read our information about inner core temperature and the importance of checking that. Because you arc doing sprint work, your inner core temp will spike.

The biggest mistake new moms or moms to be say is, "Well, yes, but won't I know when I'm too hot?" No. You cannot judge how hot you are by the amount you sweat.

The only red flag is see is the plyometrics and jumping rope. Again, you are conditioned. But the impact may be a little too much. Personally, I did high impact/plyo workout the first trimester and, as long as I watched my inner core temp -- was fine. But do you really need to continue jumping rope?? This is a personal choice but I would probably move away from that. As you grow through the pregnancy, you will need to stop the jumping.

The tai Chi and Pilates are also wonderful, wonderful exercises to help relief stress, elongated muscles, build/help flexibility and static strength. But they can be very stressful and generate high inner core temperatures. Because you are conditioned, this should not be a problem as long as you watch the inner core temp and stay hydrated. However, during the latter half of your second trimester, these stretches may become a little too intense as your joints begin to loosen. As an athlete, you will know when to scale back. By your second trimester, really listen to your body. If you do not enjoy the stretches as you once did, skip it. It's okay!!!

You will continue your Nordic track work and walking (which you can add light hand weights to) for a strong cardio workout.

The weight lifting looks great!! Keep it up! But I would ask that you invest the money to see a trainer at least once a month -- just to be sure that you maintain a good form while your body changes. Many athletes do not realize how much they adjust/change/shift while lifting weights when they are pregnant. Because you are adjusting to the ever expanding tummy, you do not realize how much you've changed your stance. So, have a professional trainer spot you, check you while your workout. It's a safety precaution to make sure you lift safely throughout the pregnancy. Otherwise, looking good.

Swimming is fabulous and highly recommended. The road bike ... I don't like. I know it's fun and offers more resistance but the chances of you being chased by a dog, run off the road, hitting gravel ... all things that cannot be controlled are a possibility that could cause harm to YOUR BABY. Therefore, I typically ask my clients to forgo the outside cycling and stick to stationary. You can create your own sprint interval training program on the bike (again, watching the inner core temp).

While you should concentrate on checking your inner core temperature, you must also stay focused on being properly hydrated. The one thing I hear pregnant clients say is, "Ugh! All I do is go to the bathroom..." For this reason, many do not drink as much water as they should. I don't care if it seems like you are going to the bathroom 17 times a day. Continue drinking (lightly) fluids while you work out. Replenish your body so that it will help your temp stay cooler. Dehydration is also a cause for morning sickness. The more hydrated you are the less likely you are to get headaches, feel nauseous, eat poorly.

If you are able/willing to see a trainer at least once a month, this person will also help assess your training schedule as your body grows. Finally, I want to say that because you are so motivated and committed ... it really is okay if at some point you say, "You know, I'm really pooped." and fall off the training schedule. Once an athlete, always an athlete. You will return to training and you will get your body back. So, no frets ... just enjoy this time.

Question:

I am a dancer (ballet and modern dance) and dance teacher. I am supposed to be performing when I will be about 10 weeks pregnant. I have taken the last few weeks off and am getting ready to start working out again. I just found out I am about three months pregnant. Do you know anything about dancing during pregnancy? There is a lot of jumping, leaping and turning involved. There are times when I can slow down and pace myself during the dances so I'm not going full out for the hour. What do you think?

Answer:

You are a conditioned athlete continuing a routine you are adjusted to. What worries most physicians is when a pregnant woman decides to take on a new sport or training routine because she is pregnant. The jumps and leaps are nothing new to you and should be able to continue dancing until you decide it just doesn't feel comfortable. Typically, I shy away from jumps with pregnant women. However, by virtue of being a dancer, your jumps/leaps are part of the dance and very much a part of your training. Unlike people who jump during a cardio bootcamp class, for example, yours is about form. However, there are some things to be considered:

You need to have your doctor's permission before continuing. Obviously, I do not know your medical history so you need to be cleared by a medical professional. You must also know that the jumps are high-impact and could pose a problem if you are a high-risk pregnancy. For this reason, you must outline what you do for your doctor and OB/GYN.

I suspect by virtue of being a professional, you will know when it's time to stop and make the proper modifications while instructing others. Most professional athletes/instructors wean themselves by the beginning of the second trimester.

Question:

"I have a question regarding dancing while being pregnant. My girlfriend is pregnant with our baby and she is a dancer at school. Is it safe for her to dance? Is it safe for her to dance Hip Hop style? I'm asking because I don't want to hurt our baby."

Answer:

You're a good man to be so concerned and involved!

Firstly, because we do not know her medical history, she really needs to see her OB/GYN to be sure that he/she knows everything. Whether your girlfriend has a family history of hypertension, diabetes, for example, this needs to be discussed. Also, her doctor needs to give her the medical permission to continue the intense dancing.

Now, having said this ... and assuming that your doctor tells her that she may continue with what she's been doing ... she should be able to continue. However, there are factors the two of you need to consider.

Right now she is in her first trimester. Her body is acclimated to the dance routines so she's not doing anything new or difficult. Outside of having nausea from 'morning sickness' (which can be all day), she can continue as normal but she MUST stay hydrated. That is, she needs to drink water throughout the day. Most American women are naturally dehydrated anyway because so many drink coca-colas or coffee rather than water. She might complain to you that now that she's pregnant ALL SHE EVER DOES is go to the bathroom. But she needs to drink water throughout the day.

Now, let's talk Hip Hop. This is very intense, demanding a great amount of energy. As a result, her inner core temperature can spike without her realizing how hot she really is until AFTER she's done dancing. If her routine is, oh, say, five minutes -- she's safe. But if she is dancing intensely for more than 20 minutes, she needs to be able to stop and take her inner core temperature. The reason is because your baby is 1 degree Celsius higher than the body temperature of your girlfriends. And, your baby has no way to sweat -- to release heat. Because of this, experts insist that female athletes/dancers must not let their own temperature exceed 101 degree F.

So, how does she check her inner core temperature??
Okay, this is kind of icky but it's the best way for you, your girlfriend to know that your baby is safe.
Go buy a rectal thermometer. After 20 minutes, your girlfriend should dance her little self to the bathroom and use the rectal thermometer to check her temp. Again, it should not go over 101 degree F.

Now, let's talk about the upcoming dance event. By this stage in her pregnancy, her body will have changed. By the second trimester, her joints will begin to soften -- getting ready for childbirth. Female athletes/dancers need to pay special attention to their changing bodies. Particularly doing something like Hip Hop -- she could twist a knee or hip because the body is preparing for childbirth. The good news is, she is strong and limber. Most likely as she moves along in her pregnancy, she will learn how NOT to move and twist and will adjust as her belly grows.
Together, there are things you can do for your baby. 1) Make sure momma is hydrated. 2) Make momma check her inner core temperature. 3) Make sure momma takes pre-natal vitamins. The biggest mistake young, active moms-to-be make is saying "I feel strong" or "I feel okay, I don't need to take vitamins." Well, guess what? Your baby will take all the nutrients he or she needs from your girlfriend and without your girlfriend realizing it, she can become anemic or depleted in other ways which will increase her chances of getting injured or sick. (If the prenatal vitamins make her stomach upset -- which is common -- have her take the vitamins with a glass of milk just before she goes to bed. She will sleep through the digestion of the pills which is what makes most women sick and the baby will thrive!!). Finally, 4) be sure that your doctor understands everything she is doing/eating/lifting/jumping/running! Think like a team.
Please keep me posted and be sure to ask more questions as she moves along in her pregnancy. Good luck! You will be a great daddy.

3. The Pros and Cons of Yoga

Today, one of the oldest forms of exercise has resurfaced with great popularity. Yoga. You may have even taken yoga without even realizing it as forms (however mild or distorted) of it appear in aerobic, dance, kickbox, and sports warm-up routines. The concept is simplistic: treat the integrated body and spirit as a whole rather than working the body as independent parts. Students of yoga learn to connect the spiritual body with the physical – all which means deep stretching and challenging poses.

For this reason, there are most certainly pros and cons to the art and exercise of yoga while pregnant.

Question:

"I'm four weeks pregnant and was wondering if I can continue to do my lotte berk and bar method workouts throughout my pregnancy? I also do "Walk Away the Pounds," Pilates, yoga, and my stationary bike. Are these safe to do?"

Answer:

All of these exercises are excellent ways to work out throughout your pregnancy if you have already acclimated to such routines. We always caution against stating something new during your pregnancy unless you are working out with a trainer. And, of course, you must speak with your physician and OB/GYN before continuing (or beginning) an exercise. Having said this, lotte berk is also a great way to reduce stress, build muscle strength (you are doing to need strength in the labor and delivery room!), and flexibility which will all help with your recovery after the baby is born.

But there are some specific exercises associated with yoga, Pilates, and lotte berk and bar method that we need to pay attention to as your pregnancy progresses. People are misguided in believing that only when you jump around to the pulsating music in an acrobics class or run for 45 minutes on the treadmill are you really burning calories. Yoga and the bar method, for example, are two of the most demanding exercises in existence. All muscles are utilized.

Your inner core temperature can soar without you ever realizing how hot you've actually become. Remember that your baby has no way of sweating or regulating his or her own body heat. This is your job.

Again, because you are acclimated to these exercises you can continue but learn to listen to your body. Pregnant women happily continue with their yoga, Pilates, and berk lotte classes throughout the duration of their pregnancies but eventually scale back on the stretches and pulls that no longer feel good.

(Read Chapter 4: What Your Trainer Isn't Telling You on checking your inner core temperature and how to properly read your pulse).

Question:

"I have been doing Bikram Yoga for several years now, 5-6 days a week. I am concerned about continuing as I just found out I am pregnant. I have read a lot about not raising your core temperature. However, there are gals doing hot yoga who are pregnant and others at the studio who say they wouldn't do it. My doctor

doesn't really seem to have an answer. Do you have any more insight or knowledge on this subject with all your years of being an athlete?"

Answer:
Here's my first response. Grrrr.

Why would anyone who knows about inner core temperature be willing to take hot yoga while pregnant?

You are smart to be asking. The answer is – don't risk it. You've been doing this intense exercise for over five years. No doubt, you are in fabulous condition and could easily handle the workload while pregnant. But this is not the issue. The real issue is inner core temperature and how it might affect your baby.

The entire principle behind hot yoga is to generate more body heat, thus allowing you to become more flexible, testing and stretching the muscles above and beyond what you might in a room temperature atmosphere. In a room where the temperature is maintained at 95-100 degrees F., this is already a problem. As the entire idea is to have a vigorous yoga session to promote profuse sweating, thereby ridding the body of toxins, puts your baby in a possibly very dangerous temperature zone.

Now is not the time to be focused on profuse sweating. Given your background, yoga is fine but stay away from the hot yoga.

Question:
"About a year ago, I started going to a Yoga studio where we practice power yoga in a heated room for a 90-minute class. I have been trying to conceive for the past three months and I am not sure if I should stop going to the studio. Can you please give me some advice?"

Answer:
Current evidence indicates that you should probably find another studio during this time of conception and pregnancy. While the correlation between caffeine, heat, stress, and pregnancy continue to be discussed and analyzed, you can bet heat/inner core temperature is tops on the list.

You inner core temperature increases significantly during power yoga sessions. If you love yoga, find a studio that continues to work your body and spirit but does not cause your inner core temperature to exceed 101 degree F.

Question:
"I love your advice! You are the first person who has made me feel ok about the intensity of my workouts.

On that note, I do have one question…I am a yoga instructor and I have a very vigorous practice that includes jumping back to chaturanga and very deep twists. Every yoga instructor I've spoken to seem to think that jumping back (and jumping forward) should not be done during the first trimester and that twists should be very gentle, if done at all.

My biggest problem has been the nausea all day, so the twists don't feel so great anyway, but my practice just doesn't seem the same without jumping back to chaturanga. What do you think? Also, I gave into pressure from friends and family and stopped running (3-5 miles) about three months ago. Would it be safe to start again even with a two month break.

Thank you so much for all your fabulous advice and support, it has been an absolute pleasure reading your answers."

Answer:

Thank you and it is women like you who inspire me. Boy, I know all about family pressure and constant questions that no one seems to be able to answer. We, as a people, are always looking forward in medicine and training yet, pregnant athletes are left behind. It is just easier to tell mothers-to-be to take the tried and true safe road.

So, this is what I would say to your family and friends who pressure you ... we KNOW that women who work out during pregnancy have faster and easier deliveries, recover more quickly, suffer less from postpartum-depression, and enjoy their pregnancies more. We KNOW that women who work out during pregnancy are more likely to eat better, sleep better, suffer less from headaches and nausea (although I have to say I was one of the ones who had terrible morning sickness in all three pregnancies), drink more water, and communicate with their OB/GYNs than women who do not work out. And, if that's not enough, we KNOW that the children of women who worked out during their pregnancies have better verbal and analytical skills, are more concise and articulate, and have lower body fat.

If that doesn't do it, you can go back to the old tried and true for YOU. That is... it makes you happy. As a yoga instructor (and by the way, I'm jealous. You guys are so cool! *secret desire to be a yoga instructor...), you are in great shape physically but you also know your body. Here is the number one rule of pregnant athletes -- do it if it feels good.

So, at 7+ weeks, as long as the jumping back is not too stressful and continues to feel good/normal, please continue. You've read my responses about inner core temperature. As a yoga enthusiast, I know this will be your greatest challenge -- that is, keeping your inner core temperature from spiking. By the jump back/twists and running may all be continued as long as you are hydrated, you feel good and your inner core temperature is safe. Again, let me emphasis that because you are a professional and know what feels right, what does not, I leave this to your discretion. I would certainly advise a newcomer to the art of yoga to stop the jumping.

In regards to running, do it if it feels good. Take it slow and easy. Enjoy it. If you find the pounding too much or that you are more out of breath than you like (a very common problem for experienced but newly pregnant athletes), stick to what you like most. Now, having said all this, be sure that your own OB/GYN knows what you are doing, how intense the workouts are, and what miles (if any) you run. While you may not always have the friends/family on board, you do want a strong baby team. This would include your doctor. Educate your family about inner core temperatures, heart rate, proper hydration and what your doctor says.

Let's All Do the Twist!!

It stands to reason that if you've perfected specific moves in yoga or almost any form of exercise that you can continue the activity while pregnant, yes? Not always. As you read about the broad and round ligaments, your body is only so flexible as you become more and more pregnant. You're not Gumby.

As your pregnancy continues, your ligaments soften and your joints loosen – all in preparation for the biggest exercise of them all – labor and delivery. Therefore, it is essential that you listen to your body, treating it with the respect it needs at this time. Heavy, deep twisting and stretching may not be what the doctor ordered.

Question:

I exercise regularly. My workouts include cardio and yoga that sometimes includes head stands, handstands, deep twisting and back bending, etc. If my husband and I are trying conceive, should I refrain from any of these activities around the possible conception period?"

Answer:

You are in great shape and have been doing these activities for some time. There is no reason for you to stop right now.

However, you may want to consider heat. If you are doing hot yoga, I would urge stepping away from this for now. Heat, stress, and caffeine can interfere with fertilization. When you do get pregnant, please let me know so we can have another talk about your contortionist acts!! Standing on your head and back bends are not recommended for the pregnant.

As always, I urge you to talk to your doctors because I do not know your medical background/history, I may not have the full picture and am unaware of certain medical conditions. In the meantime, while you are worrying about your physical routines, be aware that what your husband does may also affect your ability to become pregnant. We know, for example, that smoking can damage sperm, as can heavier use of alcohol, dehydration, and heat.

Question:

"I have just found out I am pregnant (maybe with twins!). I regularly participate in power yoga and Pilates. How long in my pregnancy can I continue with Pilates and power yoga (my gym does not offer prenatal equivalent classes)?"

Answer:

Twins! Double the pleasure, not the workout or food! Congrats! And, yes, you will want to be in shape for those babies. As a regular yoga and Pilates student, you may certainly continue your exercise program -- with a few rules. You must get a thumbs-up from your OB/GYN. Be sure that s/he knows exactly what your exercise routine is and your current health statistics. Remember that as your pregnancy progresses, your body composition will change -- ligaments and pelvic joints are stretching and loosening in preparation for childbirth. This is NOT a time to stretch to the extreme. As your yoga instructor coos, "No pain, no gain..." you can happily beg off. Thousands of studies have been conducted on female athletes during their pregnancy and found that yoga/stretching routines are most beneficial to labor and delivery, including a faster recovery after baby -- in your case babies -- are born. But, because your joints do loosen, do not press yourself too hard. Enjoy the exercise, stay limber, stretch those muscles (yes, you can feel the burn) but within reason. You have been doing yoga long enough, you know what feels good and what doesn't.

But we have a problem with the POWER of yoga. I would strongly urge you to find a regular yoga class. There is no need at this point in your life to take power yoga classes. Happily, you've already laid the groundwork for an exercise routine. No doubt, your muscles are strong and supple. With a regular yoga class, you can continue to stretch and work the muscles without overeating or stressing your joints.

Be sure to talk to your instructor and makes sure s/he is qualified to instruct pregnant athletes. Finally, enjoy. This may be the last time you get to work out in peace and quiet for a while!!!!

Question:

"I am so bummed. I just started doing yoga and love it. I have never liked exercise before but I love this. Then, I just found out I am pregnant. I can't keep doing all the stretching and deep twists, can I?"

Answer:

Of course you can!

Ahh, but let me qualify this answer. You've mentioned that yoga is relatively new to you so many of the moves are foreign to you/your muscles. There is no need to do the deep twists. Modify.

Any instructor worth his or her salt will not only understand this but can give you alternative moves. Be sure to tell your instructor that you are pregnant. Of course, you need to get medical permission before continuing.

You can make special requests of your students. When I train, it seems that I always have a student that needs some special tweaking. Someone has a bad knee, is pregnant, coming back from a car accident … any good trainer can direct his or her class to do one thing, then turn to you and say, "Okay, you need to do this …" But your instructor can't help you modify moves if he or she doesn't know you're pregnant. Talk to your trainers!

*If you think you would like to try yoga and are now pregnant, there are no rules against it. Of course, you must get medical permission. But you can and should check out "beginner" yoga videos at library. Before investing in a class or getting in over your head, take some time to review a beginner's yoga video and see if this is something you might be able to do. Gentle stretching and breathing exercises can be a great prenatal exercise for you.

Can Yoga Benefit Baby?

While hot yoga is a no-no, yoga can be a wonderful exercise for your baby. Studies have shown that women who study yoga are less likely to have pregnancy-related hypertension and premature labor. Researchers in India and the United States found that women who practiced yoga an hour a day fared better than those who walked (30 minutes, twice daily).

It is believed that yoga increases the blood flow to the baby, also limiting the mother's stress hormones. And yes, babies can and do react from momma's stress hormones.

Question:
Help! I live up in the mountains where, on a nice day, I can push my toddler in the stroller but in bad weather (pretty much over half the year) I'm locked in the house. Now that I'm pregnant, I can imagine I'm going to balloon. What can I do that I don't have to stop a dozen times because my toddler is doing something he's not supposed to? Help!"

Answer:
Try Momma and Toddler yoga!
Yoga can be as fun for your son as it is beneficial to you. From warrior and sun salutation to bridge and dancer's pose, the two of you can work on balance, stretching, breathing, and bonding together. What could be better!
Take a trip to the library to find a video for beginners and together, giggle and stretch your way through a great workout. You will be amazed how quickly your son will take to the exercise and love this special time with momma. I am frequently told stories of how toddlers/small children actively seek out their mothers, "Okay, it's time to work out now!"

Prenatal Yoga

If you really want to do yoga or you already practice it, why not give prenatal yoga a chance? Don't delude yourself into thinking a prenatal class would not challenge you. This is a great class for you and your baby. Prenatal teaches poses, breathing cues and helps prepare you for the big day. This yoga will help you both physically and emotionally during labor.

4. The Joys of Walking and Swimming

Hippocrates once said, "Walking is man's best medicine." Okay, so he didn't specifically mention pregnant women but you'll be pleased to know just what great medicine walking is for a mother-to-be. Both swimming and walking are low-impact forms of exercise that offer a long list of benefits from improving muscle tone, stamina, and metabolism to reducing levels of bad cholesterol and anxiety.

Let's discuss walking first.

Do you remember when they taught Mr. Freeze Meister to walk? Don't remember? Oh, come on. It was when Mother Nature's sons, Mr. Freeze Meister and Mr. Heat Meister, tried to stop Christmas and Mrs. Claus went to reason with them. Mrs. Claus quickly figured out Mr. Freeze Meister was crabby because he really couldn't get around. So, she and her helpful elves began singing to him, "Just put one foot in front of the other... and soon you'll be walking out the door." It was totally irresponsible of them. They had no idea what they were talking about and . . .did you see him? He looked as though he might topple over any second. His brother, the Heat Meister, on the other hand, was a ball of fire. Literally. He was on the balls of his feet, bouncing around with his warmed muscles. He was ready for the 100-mile walk-off.

Don't believe me? This holiday season, check out the vintage cartoon. Mr. Freeze Meister is clearly walking – if you can call it that – flat footed. Good walking or running form is essential to better, stronger strides; easier on your joints and, in the long run, will help burn more calories/fat.

So, how do you walk? If you are walking flat footed (meaning the entire underside of your foot land evenly on the pavement), chances are you are moving at a leisurely pace and too slowly to really benefit. This is very hard on your knees, hips and lower back. Try walking so that the heels of your feet hit first. Land lightly on the heels and roll forward on your foot, pushing off the ground with your toes. In this position, your calf muscles are already poised, ready to push off another strong stride. By doing this, you may need to shorten your walk a little as you adjust to the harder workout. Yes, you are burning more fat and will have a higher heart rate because you are having to work more. Stand straight; keep your arms and wrists loose. Most people want to walk with clenched fists but you will benefit more if your upper body is relaxed, allowing your arms to swing back and forth, thus working upper body as well.

If running, keep your position tall and remain on the balls of your feet for the entire job. Again, this is easier on the joints and will increase your stamina tenfold.

You know, Mr. Freeze Meister and Mr. Heat Meister were brothers and yet, Mr. Freeze Meister looked a hundred years older than his brother. Coincidence? I think not! It's all in the way you walk!

Question:

"I am about four weeks right now and I was wondering if I could start walking every day. I have been active in the past, lifting weights and running about 2-3 times a week. However, I hurt my back this summer and have been unable to do very much. I was just getting back in the groove when I found out I was pregnant. Can I or should I walk?"

Answer:

Finding your groove is important—especially when you are pregnant. I would say "yes" to walking but you must first see your physician. Questions arise as to how you injured your back and if you've been properly treated. Are you doing physical therapy? I don't know what damage has been done to your back and am concerned about possible back injury or aches later in your pregnancy.

For a moment, let's assume that your back injury was only temporary and you've fully recovered walking is an excellent way to stay fit and, in your case, slowly move back into exercise with low impact stress. If the injury was indeed temporary and you've fully recovered, you should be able to go right back to your old walking routine (with medical permission). But if you're injury is on-going (however tolerable), we need to address it now. As your body grows, more and more pressure will be put on your back. Before you entertain walking, before you consider lifting weights, speak to your doctor about seeing a physical therapist. A good therapist will not only help you rebuild the back, address the injuries, but set you up with a strong wellness/fitness program.

Question:

"I have started a "Walk Away the Pounds" exercise video that is a moderate walking exercise program that doesn't really include anything strenuous. You just walk a mile in 20 minutes. I haven't really done any exercise since college. I have had two easy, successful pregnancies. I am now pregnant with my third. I'm in my second trimester and want to know if it is okay to do this video once or twice a week?"

Answer:

Absolutely . . . but this is contingent upon your physician's approval. If you have been working out to this video and feel strong, happy doing so, then keep on walking. The important thing here is to listen to your body. You've had two healthy, "easy" pregnancies prior to this pregnancy. You know what feels right, what does not. Walking really is one of the best things you can do while you are pregnant. In fact, when pregnant you can do much more than walk but it is all based on your personal workout routine and desires.

At this point in your life, do what makes you happy. I want you to feel energized after and because of your workouts.

Remember to check your inner core temperature if/when the weather is hot or you've gone beyond the 20 minutes of walking. Stay hydrated and be sure to walk with a buddy. If you decide you want to increase the workout and make your workouts just a bit more challenging, add 1-2 pound hand weights to tone your arms and raise your heart rate ever so slightly.

Question:
"I am 3 to 4 weeks pregnant now. Before being pregnant I didn't do any exercise or sport, because I was studying and didn't have time for it. Only in the evenings I walked one, two hours almost every day. I was going to start swimming but I have just discovered that I am pregnant. I also have back pains very often. Is it wise to start swimming now, or I should only continue walking while I am pregnant?"

Answer:
Congrats! And I am glad you are thinking about exercise, particularly because you already have a back problem. It is important to build a strong core (abs/back) as pregnancy can put stress on your back (both upper and lower). Having said this, however, I cannot advise jumping into the pool just yet.

You need to speak with your doctor on two counts. First, you need to have a medical clearance regarding overall health. Then, you need to address your back pains. Is this from an injury? Is it your spine? Or muscular?

Swimming is a great exercise for both pregnancy and injury but you may very well need physical therapy before exercising on your own. Speak to your doctor about your injury/pain and working with a physical therapist. Typically, I would be very excited about you beginning a swimming program to compliment your walking -- great exercises -- but I worry about the back issue. Be smart, make an appointment with your doctor, and make sure everything is okay before you start anything.

Let's also talk about the walking. While walking is also a fabulous exercise, the compression or strain on your injured/inflamed back could only worsen the problem. So, we want to be safe. Speak to your doctor about how long you've been walking. Do you walk with weights? Or with your dog (who pulls or tugs hard on the leash)? Do you push a stroller? What kind of shoes are you wearing?

Once you have clearance to swim and walk, put yourself on a regular program so that your body can become acclimated to something. Your safest route is to speak with a trainer who can assess your current fitness level. But you can begin walking or swimming (with medical permission) slowly and build your time and distance as you become more conditioned.

Walking Tall

Posture is everything. When you are walking, be sure to keep your head up and back elongated but relaxed. Pump the arms and walk with purpose!

Question:
"If I've never really done anything before (okay, I'm a total couch potato), how do I know how long or far I should start walking? I really want to start doing something but don't know how much I can do."

Answer:
Ahh, my little couch potato. You know what I'm going to say … please talk to your doctor first. Because I do not know your medical history, I want to be sure you are safe before taking on anything new. Once you've been given the green light, invest in good walking shoes. I know there is the desire to just get something cheap but don't. Your feet will ALSO change during pregnancy so let's take good care of them. Think of this as an investment for the future.

Get out that journal and begin to record the last days of your couch potato ways! Start by walking three times a week. These walks can be anywhere from 10 – 20 minutes. Record your distance, time, and how you felt. Be sure to include the time of day as you may discover different times of the day where your energy level peaks.

My own journal might look something like this:

Week 1:

Monday	12 minutes/0.8 mile.
Tuesday	off
Wednesday	12 minutes/0.8 mile
Thursday	off
Friday	14 minute/0.9 mile
Saturday	off

*If you feel strong enough to add to the walking routine, add another day to the next week but do not add too much distance/time just yet. Don't become overly enthusiastic until you know you can handle the program.

Week 2:
  Monday   12 minutes
  Tuesday   12 minutes
  Wednesday off
  Thursday   14 minutes
  Friday   12 minutes
  Saturday   off

*If you felt great in week 2 -- continue on.

Week 3:
  Monday   14 minutes
  Tuesday   12 minutes
  Wednesday off
  Thursday   14 minutes
  Friday   12 minutes
  Saturday   10 minutes

Slowly build until you are comfortably walking 20 minutes/five days a week. At this point, if you feel you want a more challenging workout – in the weeks to come but DO NOT rush this program – add 1-2 pound hand weights.

Be sure to record how you feel during and after the walks, what you've eaten, how much water you have taken in, and how your feet feel. Check your inner core temperature and be sure to walk with a buddy!

Question:
 "My mother-in-law says I'm not supposed to walk more than 1 mile. But I've been walking for years and have even done a couple of competitive race walks. I'm not exactly Olympic material but I can't stand the idea of only walking a mile! Is that true?"

Answer:
 No. If you've been walking 45 minutes to an hour at a competitive pace, you may continue this routine. But we may need to tweak your routine. Like a runner, you should only have one long walk. Put your competitive shoes away for now and focus on breathing and form rather than speed and times.
 Focus on more of a soft-strike when your heel hits the ground rather than the hard strike competitive race walkers can have.
 You may walk five, even six days a week but remember that speed is not on the agenda. Grab a buddy and enjoy your walks. (See the story of Michelle Rohl).

Swimming

Question:
"I am 24 weeks and I'm starting to swim. Could you recommend me some basic exercises that I should do before, during and after I swim?"

Answer:
As always, we ask that you speak to your physician first. Because we do not know your medical history, it is imperative that you and your OB/GYN are on the same page and that s/he understands what you want to do for an exercise routine. This should include how often you will swim. Having said this, let's assume that your doctor tells you that you are cleared for an exercise routine that includes swimming.

My first recommendation is to sit with a personal trainer -- I know that this cost money but it really is worth your while to meet with a trainer just once to have a personal assessment done. We need to know what you can do. If, for example, you are or were a completely sedentary person, I would suggest 15 to 30 minutes of swimming for three days a week in which you try to build your cardio -- meaning, taking less resting breaks between laps. However, if you have some walking/running/aerobic background, a trainer can help you with an exercise routine that will allow you to go for greater distances and build endurance.

Swimming is an excellent exercise for pregnant women as it is wonderful for the joints. It is low-impact yet allows your endurance and muscle core to be worked. You should have one day of swim where you have a half play day -- swimming around for 15 minutes. This is your warm-up. Then, set out for laps. Again, this is difficult because I do not know your physical conditioning. Talk to a trainer. You can set up goals for yourself – for example: 20 laps in 30 minutes or 30 laps in 30 minutes. As you work to make or beat this goal, you also work on form. The beauty? You can do this throughout your pregnancy and be ready for the biggest athletic event of your life ... child labor.

Two days in the pool should be spent with, if possible, water aerobics. This is a wonderful exercise. Unfortunately, a lot of people snub this because they see older or obese people in the pool and think it can't be challenging. Wrong!!! It's great and will benefit you greatly. Again, it will allow you to work with and talk to a trainer. This is three days of work out (in the water.) Now, add one day in the gym for circuit training -- again, if possible. Why do you want to do this if you are already working out in the pool?? While walking, running, aerobics, or swimming are great, you need to add some weight work to your routine.

Light weights!! Again, working with a trainer, even once, will help you learn form, the proper weights to use, and how to most benefit your muscle core/body. The muscles women report to be the most sore or fatigued after childbirth are the back, shoulders, bicep/triceps and calves. These are also the most neglected by most women. We are so focused on our legs, we forget these other muscles. By

140

swimming laps, working a light routine on the circuit and water aerobics, you will hit everything and feel great.

Like so many mothers-to-be, U.S. gold-medalist swimmer Angel Martino wondered how much exercise was too much. She wasn't the least bit concerned about her diet or gaining weight, putting on 50 pounds. "I wanted to gain weight because I think the baby is happier and healthier that way. Because I am an athlete, I knew I would be able to lose it." The real question for her was, how much could she train.

The six-time gold medalist trained in the pool throughout her pregnancy, but it wasn't always easy. When I first spoke to her and her coach/husband, Mike, they were concerned because even as an Olympic athlete, the conventional thinking was always …"stay at 140 beats per minute." For Angel, this was nothing but "just to be safe, we would hover around that 140," says Mike.

Because she was already in great shape, holding at 140 bpm felt more like a warm-up. Finally, they realized that she was happier when she swam at a pace that "felt right." For Angel, a world renowned athlete, she would allow her heart rate to go up to 180 for two laps. Then, she would take a few cool down laps to let her heart rate go back to 140. Again, she would swim hard, repeating the process for an hour-long workout.

While you may never see the Olympic Games, you may adopt the philosophy of swimming to what "feels right," if you are already a regular swimmer. Swimming in this manner will keep you strong, your muscles viable, heart healthier and disposition happier. When Momma is happy, baby is happy!

As for Angel, she swam 2 ½ miles the day before she gave birth but for her, this was a mild workout. As her pregnancy progressed, she gradually scaled down the number of laps and swam for pure enjoyment.

Question:
"My husband and I are currently trying to get pregnant. I have been a swimmer all my life. I mainly do freestyle and butterfly. I have two questions. Will I be able to continue to do flip turns once I am pregnant and through the entire pregnancy. Will I be able to continue to swim butterfly?"

Answer:
In regards to the flips, your body will answer this question for you. You may continue to do the flips easily in the first trimester but as your body changes, you will most likely discover this no longer feels good. Olympic swimmers often forgo the flips during pregnancy believing there is no need to perfect this technique when the swimmers physique is gone. You will have plenty of time for this later. It is strongly suggested that you simply enjoy the swim.

The same rules apply for butterfly. Because this is such an exhausting and demanding style, your heart rate will be elevated. The good news is, you are already in great shape but I want you to focus on the enjoyment of swimming rather than times once you enter your second trimester.

Your first move? Once you learn you are pregnant, talk to your doctor and OB/GYN to be sure everyone is in the same boat – or pool.

Question:
"Should I be worried about the chlorine in the pool?"

Answer:
Good news. The opposite is true. The chlorine will actually help protect you and your baby against disease-causing bacteria. All too often, gym equipment can carry more organisms that you or I want to think about … all those sweaty bodies! The pool offers a sanitary (when properly managed) workout environment.

Even better, for women who experience swollen feet/ankles, lower back pain, and aching hips, swimming and water aerobics is a great way to exercise without weight bearing stress.

Just as you would with walking or running, keep an active journal, writing down the times you started, how many laps you did and how you felt. Be sure to include your nutritional diet and any other activities to be shared with your doctor. You will see the typical peaks and valleys of training.

5. Weight Lifting and Circuit Training

Question:
Why is it bad to lift heavy things when pregnant? How heavy is considered too heavy?

Answer:
A great question and, until recently, one that few people knew the real answers to. In the past, it has always been standard procedure to caution pregnant women from lifting anything heavy because it stood to reason that the strain might not be good for the baby. Over time, we learned that as you move along in your pregnancy, your joints soften/shift preparing for childbirth. The new concern was that heavy weight could cause injury to both mother and baby.

To compound this, many women report feeling clumsier. Again, this is not a time to be lifting heavy objects.

But within the last decade, a new question was posed. For athletic women, for women who are used to lifting heavy weight, is this still a problem? And for many OB/GYN's, this was a head scratcher. Just as we advise women in exercise, women are advice to stay away from lifting heavy items (or beginning a new exercise routine) because it's assumed this is an activity you are not used to. But what if you are acclimated to lifting 100 lbs bags??

The United States Olympic Committee and International Olympic Committee funded a study to see how elite athletes fared during pregnancy as they continued with their training -- including lifting heavy objects. Note that these are women who are completely and totally acclimated to a specific training program.

The result did not surprise the elite athletes. They were able to continue their training -- including heavy lifting -- until the second trimester. At this point, some women stopped because they felt pressured by family to stop while others did have injuries (while none were documented to do with the training). By the third trimester, more women stopped intense exercise because they were simply tired or reported that lifting just didn't feel good. But the end result was: exercise (or lift) to comfort.

Now, where does this leave you? Not knowing your medical and exercise background, we have to insist that you speak to your OB/GYN. This is a must. And, when you speak to him or her, you must be sports specific -- that is, tell him/her exactly what you intend to lift -- how much, how often.

Secondly, you really should work with a personal trainer who will teach you HOW to lift. Form is everything and you really can prevent injuries by working with someone. Do not forget that your body will be ever changing which means what works well this month may have to be tweaked, altered, changed next month.

Do not try anything new. Do not try to "show someone" how strong you can continue to be during your pregnancy. Always, always, always.. your health and that of your baby must be your number one concern.

For many, this continues to be a question to ponder. How much is too much? The answer has everything to do with your activity level prior to pregnancy. For regular exercisers, women who have committed themselves to the gym, they already have a fair idea of what and how much they can lift, squat, lunge, curl, and pull. For them, the answer is simple: stick to the already existing exercise plan and modify as the pregnancy moves along. This is not a time for a gym novice to begin a weight lifting program!

*If you have never lifted weights before, you must first speak with your physician and a certified trainer. Do not attempt to create an exercise program with weights for yourself by yourself!

But let's be clear: weight lifting is great for the body. We're not talking about squatting 400 pounds. Light weights can do wonders for you and your body as it progresses through the pregnancy. Suddenly, your upper and middle trapezoids (back of the shoulder) are aching from the pull of your heavier breasts. You feel like you are dragging, sapped of strength and energy. The solution? Weight lifting and a reasonable cardio routine.

Question:
"I've heard that it is good for you to work out with light weights and higher repetitions during pregnancy but I'm not exactly sure what I'm supposed to do. Can you help?"

Answer:
You are right. You will feel so much better if you work with light weights to help build a stronger back, arms, and legs. Do not go it alone. Be sure to work with a trainer to be sure that your body position, movements, and choice of equipment/weights are safe during your pregnancy.

Just as you need to get medical permission, check your inner core temperature and heart rate, and stay hydrated, there are rules of the gym for a pregnant woman:

- Be conscious of how hard you are working. Refer back to Chapter Four: What Your Trainer Isn't Telling You. Be sure to inhale and exhale properly while lifting.
- Between sets, give yourself a longer period to recover after completing a set of repetitions. This will help both your breathing and to regulate your inner core temperature.
- Do not work for muscular failure – a weight lifting principal where you cannot do another repetition because your muscles are so fatigued.
- Do not work out, lying flat on your back. The theory is that while in a declined position blood flow to the uterus is decreased.
- Stick to the controlled exercises (machines) rather than heavier free weights. While 2-, 4-, 6-, 8-, and 10-pound weights are fine to work with, you may feel unstable with heavier weights. As your joints loosen during pregnancy, ligaments and tendons are more likely to be injured with heavy, free-weights. The machines offer stability and safety.

Typically, women who are pregnant are told to stay away from heavy lifting. This is for a number of reasons. Most women do NOT lift heavy objects, therefore, they are not used to the strain. But the norm of thinking is that pregnant women can continue exercise if it is one that her body is adjusted to. If you were to tell me that you ran, sprinted, jumped on a trampoline or cycled, I would tell you it was safe to continue as you are already acclimated to that routine.

Obviously, as your body changes, so does the routine and you are forced to re-adjust your activity. In the case of heavy lifting, we have to be very careful. What constitutes as heavy? Are you lifting 50 or 60 pounds? It is safe for you to continue this if:

1) You have your doctor's permission. Because we do not know your medical background, it is dangerous for us to say 'yes' without questioning your medical history.

2) You are lifting correctly. Again, we may assume you know how to lift as you do it all the time. However, people normally have poor form when lifting and this causes back injury. While you will most likely not hurt the baby in the least bit, an injured back could result in mandatory bed rest for you.

   The easy answer would be to say, 'yes, you may continue lifting until it is uncomfortable.' However, there are these outside factors to consider.

We suggest you find out if you are pregnant or not. With your doctors' permission, you may continue to lift the reasonable amount of weight you have been thus far but listen to your body. If you are grunting and holding your breath while lifting, stop. Be sure to lift from the legs, always starting from a squat position. Do not lean forward, pulling from the back.

The good news is your body is incredibly resilient and your body is very well protected. Other things to be concerned about -- more so than the heavy lifting -- is making sure you are properly hydrated (drink lots of water!) and that you not get too hot. Check our web for information about inner core temperature.

In regards to exercise, there are many exercises you can do. However, it is difficult to know how to guide you until we know what kind of exercise you have done in the past. If you are a walker or jogger, you may continue these activities. But if you have not done these cardiovascular workouts, we need for you to begin slowly and safely. Once again, be sure to get a medical release from your physician. Once you have done that and he or she believes it is safe for you to exercise, you can start with walking, slowly building on the time and speed in which you walk. It is highly recommended that you start with a trainer. This is someone who can talk to you about your heart rate, distance, proper form and setting goals. Of course, we know this is not always feasible, so let's take this step-by-step.

Find out if you are pregnant, talk to your doctor and then get back to us with the results. Be sure to include what kinds of workouts you have done in the past so we know what your body can handle as you begin a new routine.

Question:
"My husband and I are pregnant and just joined a gym. I know I have some weight to lose going into the pregnancy so I definitely don't want to blow up. We've joined a gym so my question is, what can I do now to help myself during the pregnancy?"

Answer:

You are already on the right track. So many of my clients come to the gym after they discover they are pregnant and appear to be worried about how their body is going to change. Good for you for being one step ahead. Now, let's get to it... yes, you are going to change during your pregnancy. The worst mistakes you can make is to delude yourself into thinking you can "control" that change. Genetics have that privilege. Some women seem to have a little ball hidden under their shirts while others balloon. All you can do is make sure you are healthy, strong, happy and accepting of what is happening.

Some would say, "Wait? You mean, it doesn't matter what I do?" No. But it is important that you not say, "I'm not going to gain more than 20 lbs during my pregnancy." You will only make yourself miserable and possibly rob yourself of proper nutrition.

First, you must talk to your physician to make sure you are given the thumbs up to continue working out. Ask about nutrition. Many OB/GYN's work with nutritionists. It is important that you take you prenatal vitamins, get the required calcium, protein and folic acid needed for you and baby. Don't fall into the trap of thinking you are eating for two. You baby takes what he or she needs from you. You need to be eating for you -- keep your muscles strong and nourished.

That leads me to your fitness question. And, yes, how well you rest and eat has direct impact on your fitness routine and fitness level. How do you train to keep your body in shape during pregnancy? Continue your training regimen but be sure you are working main muscle groups. Alternate days, working upper body one day, lower body the next day while you continue a cardio workout. Upper body strength is very important because 10 months from now when you are being asked to push, you need to have the upper body strength to grip the railing of the bed and push. You need to have stamina and endurance. Many women have c-sections simply because they have nothing left to give.

As your pregnancy moves along, you should continue working upper and lower body, combined with cardio but you can and will need to modify as your body changes. I implore you to work with a personal trainer at least once a month, every month just to have someone check your body position and workload. If you can afford a personal trainer for all workouts, that is best.

The two most neglected muscles during pregnancy? Lower back and abs. Yes, you can work those muscles. My clients who worked faithfully throughout the pregnancy, even days before giving birth had faster, easier deliveries and returned to their workouts and pre-baby body shape more quickly than those who worked out only once a week. While genetics may have its own idea how big or swollen you get, you can better determine how the pregnancy will feel and how quickly you will recover by how you eat and workout.

Question:

"I have been very active as far as exercise for about eight years. I had my son 18 months ago and resumed a VERY active routine since he was six months old. I work out six times a week. I do an hour of cardio and weight train for about 45 minutes, six times a week. I was wondering a few things. 1) Can I continue this now that I am four weeks pregnant? My heart rate range was at the high end of 170. What can it be now? My leg routine consisted of squats, lunges, and Pilates. Can I still perform these? I remember during one of my child birth classes with my son the lady mentioning not doing squats till you are 37 weeks because you will push the baby down and delivery early but they have been a part of my routine forever. My doctor will not be seeing me until next month and I am at a loss at what to do . . ."

Answer:

Good news for you. Because you are a dedicated athlete/gym rat, and because your body is acclimated to rigorous routines, you may continue. However, we have some conditions:

1) You must see your OB/GYN and let him/her know what your routine is. Because we do not know your medical history, we must insist that your doctor review your current health and workout routine to determine what is safe and what is not. From this point, I will work from the base that you have been given medical clearance to work out.

2) Stay hydrated. It seems reasonable but you would be amazed how many pregnant women (or any women for that matter) are medically dehydrated. I know, I know... all you're doing is going to the bathroom as it is but you need to drink plenty of water. Stay away from the soda pops and coffee.

3) Heart rate: You can have an elevated heart rate while working out.

HOWEVER it must not stay elevated for prolonged periods of time. I noted that your heart rate has been at the high end of 170 bpm. Again, I would caution you to watch this and be sure that you do not stay elevated for long. Talk to your doctor about this and do not be surprised if he suggests you bring this down. But please note that it does not have to be the formatted 140 bpm. As a conditioned athlete, you are beyond this point.

4) Train with a buddy. In the book **Entering the Mother Zone: Balancing Self, Health, and Family** (Wish Publishing, 2000), you can read about the relationships and benefits of training with a partner, in addition to how elite/Olympic athletes trained. (Copies of this book can be found on www.pregnancy.org)

5) Squats. Until recently, there was very little research on heavy weight bearing activities while pregnant because the safe rule of thumb was ... don't lift anything heavy. I still use this rule for new clients because it is unsafe to introduce anything new when pregnant. However, you are already used to this activity. So, having

been given permission from your doctor, you can continue the squats but lighten the load. You should not be squatting for power or to build muscle. At this point, the only reason for squatting is maintenance. For this reason, most elite athletes opt not to squat.

I suggest seat squats rather than standing. I suggest a trainer work with you and remind yourself again and again that it is OKAY to lighten the weights. While you want to feel the burn in your legs/glutes, this should not be a stressful activity for the lower back/abs. Again, use caution. Talk to your OB/GYN and trainer. Because I do not know how much you have been squatting, this is tricky business. Better to be safe than sorry.

6) Lunges. The biggest concern with lunges is that as your body changes and joints soften (in preparation of giving birth) women can injure knees and ankles during this activity. I did lunge -- however, I monitored the weights and continued to lighten then as I moved through my pregnancy.

7) Pilates and yoga. These are terrific activities in terms of lengthening muscles and staying limber. However, because they are so demanding, they are also two activities where your inner core temp can really spike without you knowing it. Several things to consider: take many water breaks, use your rectal thermometer. Talk to the instructor about inner core temp and be sure he/she knows why you are taking breaks. (For one thing, this is a great opportunity to educate more people about inner core temp!). And, monitor your movements and how deeply you stretch/train as your body changes.

So, you cannot see your doctor for another month …. With the information that I've given you, you know your body best. You know what you can do, the state of your health, and how to exercise. The biggest thing I can say at this point is, use common sense. If you feel strong -- fabulous! Have a workout that feels right. You will know when it is too much. Until you see your doctor, be sure to use the rectal thermometer, drink fluids, talk to a trainer, and perhaps lighten (or skip) the squats until you have the appointment.

So, why do you need to bring down the heart rate?

Here's the reason, as your heart rate soars, your body demands more blood/oxygen. Studies have shown that when your heart rate goes up (and stays up), baby's heart rate can go down. So, here is where interval training comes in. I would do sprint sets on the vertical climb, bike, and/or Stairmaster. Even when running stadium bleachers, I would run up, walk down.

You will note that I was training throughout my pregnancy. Your intensity WILL change as your baby grows. This is to be expected. One of the biggest and most dangerous mistakes I have seen over the years is when a competitive athlete refuses to acknowledge this and is more worried about "falling behind" in an exercise routine. Listen to your body. When your body/baby wants you to lighten the intensity -- go for it.

I've done several articles on the topic of muscle memory. In short, after baby is born, your body will return to athlete form through muscle memory.

*Another note: I cannot tell you how many athletes later report that they are stronger, more fit, more determined as mother athletes. ... hurray!

Chapter Ten
Working Outdoors

Fresh air (if you don't live around cement plants), wide open spaces, safe bike paths, trees, and a gentle breeze. What could be better for you and the baby? But exercise outside can be hazardous if you are not prepared. And just because you are getting fresh air doesn't always mean the activities you are engaged in are safe for your baby. Or you. Throughout the book, one of the recurring themes has been to use common sense. You've read testimonials from elite athletes who worried about "losing their competitive edge" yet chose the safer route while pregnant.

When you plan your outdoor activities, consider safety, weather, dogs, the intensity of your sport, and whether it is right for you at this time in your life. Above all else, have fun.

1. Know the Elements

Consider weather (severe heat or cold) before setting out. Dress appropriately. Check the website to see what kind of air quality you are having in your area. Pack water, a rectal thermometer, cell phone, and stopwatch to time your heart rate. You've thought of everything, right? But have you considered what might happen if you were charged by a dog, for example, while pushing your toddler in a stroller? Or, perhaps you've decided to take your own Fido with you.

Jogging/Walking, Dogs and Baby Strollers

It's a beautiful day and you've decided to try out your new jogging stroller with baby and dog in tow. Before your baby came along, you and your furry friend logged countless miles jogging or walking around the neighborhood. Your dog has proven to be an excellent jogging partner so you have no worries about adding a jogging stroller to the mix now that your baby is here. After all, it's a great workout for all of you, right?

As a dog trainer for more than two decades (before bobsledding. It's a long story … for another time), I cannot tell you how many times (human) clients have come in with sprained or broken ankles/wrists, scraped knees and aching bodies after colliding with their dog while jogging. Most often these injuries occur with an untrained pet but even the best of dogs can have less than stellar moments on the daily jog. A squirrel suddenly darting across your path, a bike appearing from nowhere or another dog can cause great harm to you and your baby. All too often, the baby stroller gets dumped over. Even if you have strapped your baby in, he or she can be hurt – head injuries being the number one concern.

You can continue to jog or walk with your dog and baby but you must adhere to certain safety guidelines. Of course, the safest way to exercise with your baby is to leave your dog at home, taking him/her for a walk later. But if you are determined to take both baby and dog at the same time, remember these golden rules:

1. The Stroller is Not a Hitching Post

Do not tie the end of the leash to the stroller. Joggers often find it cumbersome to handle both the stroller and lead, and decide to tie the leash to the stroller, believing they can handle the stroller better. More stroller/jogging accidents have been reported as a result of this technique than any other. While you are jogging along, your dog is searching for squirrels, cats, even blowing leaves that you might not notice until it is too late. To not hitch your dog to the stroller.

2. Wrist-Free Jogging and Walking

In the terrible event that another dog attacks you or your dog suddenly lunges forward, you must have complete control over the stroller. Many runners like to loop the handle of the leash around their wrist – again, thinking they have better control over the stroller. But if and when a runner is pulled off balance, the stroller can be knocked over. Even worse, the runner is pulled away from the stroller. It only takes a few seconds for the stroller to roll out into the street.

3. Attacked!

It is every jogger's nightmare. The only thing that could be worse than being charged by an unfriendly dog is to have your dog and baby with you. Remain calm. Pull your dog in close, stop running and use your voice. "No!" Tell the on-coming dog "No!" repeatedly, careful not to scream or shriek (as this will only excite the dog). Most dogs are people-friendly and do not wish to cause you any harm. Most likely, they are protecting a territory and simply want you to move away. Walk calmly, keeping your dog close and continue to reassure the other dog you mean no harm but you are in control. "No!" Usually, the dog will continue to bark, perhaps a little less aggressively, but will drop back, waiting for you to leave. However, there are instances in which the dog is clearly dog aggressive. He may not even notice you standing there as he is so focused on your dog. If attack is eminent, you must let your dog go. Never mind the huge danger factor of having a dogfight on top of your child, your dog will have no chance to defend him or herself if tethered to you. By letting your dog go free, you will all have a better chance of getting out of that dangerous territory safely and quickly. Again, most dogs drop back and will return to defend their turf. Your dog will either fight back or (we hope) run. Either way, this is safer for dog, owner and baby.

Even if the three of you escape unscathed, you must report this incident to the authorities. To ensure the safety of others and your next outing, the owners of the dog must be notified and warned about their dog's aggressive behavior.

4. Attacked and Alone

If you are going to be charged, it is better that you don't have a toddler with you but you are still pregnant and very much alone. The rules still apply. Do not scream, wave your arms frantically, or attempt to run. Remain calm, using the same rules stated above.

Again, report this incident.

2. Jogging and Walking

Nothing has changed from Chapter 9: The Treadmill and The Joys of Walking. As you have read, there are certain cons to using the treadmill later in your pregnancy as fitness experts worry about a misplaced foot or losing balance. But, again, we also worry about cars, wayward cyclists, charging dogs, and poor weather as you set out to exercise.

- Choose a well-lit path to walk or jog.
- Do not exercise alone.
- If you can only walk or jog during pre-dawn or dusk hours, use the treadmill.
- Do not walk your dog alone during your last trimester if he or she pulls.
- If you push a stroller, do join a stroller class. Yes, they do exist. Try www.StrollerFit.com or www.strollercize.com or www.strollerstrides.com for more information.
- Check www.airnow.gov for your local forecasts.
- Check your inner core temperature
- Bring water
- Do not wear headphones/ear pieces if you are alone.

So, what is a good walking program outside? Of course, before you begin, be sure you are cleared to do so with your doctor. The next step will be to determine how far you can walk. Here is a 30-minute sample that can/should be tweaked to best fit you. Remember, it should be challenging, not exhausting.

5 minutes	Warm up. Take a nice easy stroll.
1 minute	Speed up, really pump your arms to get your heart rate flowing. (If this is not enough, add hand weights)

4 minutes	Slow down a little, walking to catch your breath. You should be able to carry on a conversation at this point. If not … stay at this level until you can talk.
2 minutes	Again, quicken the pace.
3 minutes	Slow down until you can speak again.
3 minutes	Repeat process – speed up…
2 minutes	slow down …
4 minutes	Speed up …
6 minutes	cool down – slow pace.

*How Fit Are You? By the Cooper Institute

Mile Time:

13:30 minutes or less	Excellent
13:31 to 16:00	Good
16:01 to 18:30	Average
18:31 to 20:00	Below Average
20:01 min or low	Low

If it is a light run you desire, this walking routine above can be used as a jogging routine or even a mix between the two, walking as a recovery and jogging on the increased speed times.

3. Hiking, Cycling, Mountain Bike Workouts, and Motorcycles

Never has there been a better example of someone wanting something so much that they forgave all common sense.

I received a question regarding hiking in high altitudes while pregnant. It was from a Scandinavian woman, who lived her entire life in the mountains and was an avid hiker. Given this information, she needed to know that most women have successful pregnancies at high elevations but babies tend to be smaller and complications with the pregnancy can arise, particularly pre-eclampsia. It is believed that this may linked to lower oxygen levels delivered to the baby. And, yes, even women who are completely acclimated to hiking could have complications. For this reason, she would have to speak to her doctor, get medical permission and make her own judgment call.

Then, the red flags started to pop up.

Her doctor had discouraged her from hiking as she was pregnant with triplets. It was a high risk pregnancy because of a previous eating disorder.

She had been told by friends, family, and her own physician not to hike but had wanted so much to stay with her current exercise routine, she was only giving partial information. Once we learned what she was eating (not enough), that she was pregnant with triplets, and had some medical issues that qualified her as a high-risk pregnancy, this was a no-brainer. No hiking.

But for the most part, hiking can be a great workout providing the conditions are right.

Question:

"I need some clarification if you can offer it. I know mountain climbing poses risks to pregnant mamas because of the decreased oxygen at higher elevations. What I need clarity with, is how high of an elevation is risky? We have a backpacking hike planned next weekend when I will be six weeks along and the only info I can get about elevation levels for this particular hike is that the trail we are on "gently gains elevation." Do you have any other info that would be helpful? If you can help at all, I would really appreciate, I have to make a decision pretty quickly."

Answer:

This is a complicated issue and here's why ...

1) If you had your doctors permission, and 2) if you are in perfect medical condition (no medical or physical problems or complications), 3) if you regularly hike this particular course (or likeness to) and 4) if you are completely and totally acclimated to the kind of physical exertion you will be experiencing during the hike, 5) if you know that your inner core temperature will not spike (please read about inner core temperature and note that you will need to be able to stop to take your inner core temp without falling behind the group), you should be able to do this at six weeks. Again, you should be able to answer 'yes' to all the above "ifs".

But if this is a new kind of exercise and you are not completely acclimated to this, I would not go. Many women experience fatigue because the blood flow and oxygen usage goes to your baby. If you are huffing and puffing, not used to this activity, the strain will be too much for both you and baby. Your heart rate will sore and inner core temperature will spike, both draining you of needed energy and the baby of proper oxygen flow and -- because the baby has no way to sweat and regulate heat -- overheat.

The old thinking used to be that you could not allow your heart rate to go over 140 beats per minute -- something that will certainly happen for a novice hiker. But today, we know it is more about inner core temperature and new activities. This is a great vexation to experts because so many women get pregnant and THEN decide to get into shape, doing exercises they have never done before.

But in your case, I am also concerned with the elevation. If you answered "yes" to the above "if" scenarios, you MUST set the pace on this hike. Do not try to keep up with others. Be sure you know and understand about inner core temperature. (If you need more information beyond what our website offers, please let me know).

Stay hydrated. No colas.

Do not go if this is a new activity -- you are not a regular hiker.

Good luck. Personally, if you are not a regular hiker, I would not go. Let us know what you decide.

***

She did. After the hike, she gave an update:

"Thank you so much for the information you provided. I did go on the hike and was very aware of my body and what was going on. I didn't mention in my original e-mail that my fitness level is very high as I am a professional fitness trainer for the Canadian Military. I made my decision based on the fact that I am fit, I feel great, aside from being a little sleepy and my strength and endurance levels are quite high. I was able to lead the group, so it was my pace that everyone else had to stay with and I didn't allow myself to get exhausted. It was very hot this weekend however, we took extra precautions to stay cool, hydrated and functional. I started out on a 2km day hike that proved to be too much for me as it was a "straight up" climb on switch back trails. I ended up returning while the rest of the group continued. I was so proud of myself that I stopped because that is not my usual way. I didn't check my core temperature but as I mentioned before, we took many precautions to stay cool. We stopped often at cool streams, soaked bandana to drape around our necks and heads and drank about 4-6 litres of water each day.

I'm glad that I did this and I really appreciate your information."

If you read her information, she did everything (almost) perfectly. I would have liked to know she checked her inner core temperature but she appeared to have things well in hand. Notice that she proudly set the pace, stopped when she wanted/needed to, and was very aware of her body. She listened and respected her body. Bravo!!

The body must work harder at a higher altitude. Factor in pregnancy and you've got a body under duress. The question is how much can your body safely and happily endure? This is not just breathing thinner air. You must factor in altitude with rate of ascent, how rocky and difficult the terrain is, the pace in which you are moving, and how far along you are in your pregnancy.

Announce that you want to hike the mountains and red flags will be thrown because in your first trimester (when risk of ectopic pregnancy or miscarriage is highest), we have to factor in the altitude, pace, your medical background and, of course, physical condition. During your last trimester, we need to consider all of these things including possible injury as your joints loosen and ligaments soften. Your body has significantly changed. Is this the time to tread uneven terrain?

Do you live in higher altitude and hiking is a way of life? Or, is your family taking a vacation and this is only your third time hiking in your life? These are important issues to consider.

If you have medical permission, are in good physical condition and health, have hiked fairly regularly, and are willing to take the kind of precautions our Canadian friend did, then you will most likely do well and have a good time. As a general rule, brief stays at altitude are not believed to have negative impact on the baby or on your health.

Question:
"I am a semi-pro mountain bike/cross rider. I'm pregnant so, obviously, I'm kind of sidelined right now. But I've been walking or hiking some of the same trails I used to make on the bikes but it takes me a long time on foot. My questions are 1) Can I hike or walk for more than two hours a day on the trails and 2) can I get on the mountain bike? What do you think about either one?"

Answer:
Right off – a "no" to the mountain biking. It's not that I doubt your physical ability or agility. To be at the level you are, you have to be in amazing condition. Both your upper and lower body must be rock solid. And it's not that you can't control the bike. However, if something were to go wrong with the bike (always a possibility – you know that!), or you should momentarily lose control of the bike, lose your balance, stray from the trail, hit a soft ground or a rock … The risks are too great. This is one of those exercises I qualify as a non-controlled exercise.

As far as the hiking goes, you sound like a good candidate for such a challenging workout but there are some things you must consider.

I'm going to start by telling you things I'm sure you are already well aware of. You must first speak to your OB/GYN and personal physician about working out. I say this to everyone. Because you are in shape, your muscles are acclimated (less chances of injury) and your cardio is good. Judging by what you do, your legs and core (lower back and abs) are already strong. Still, we need to be safe and consider fetal strain as you are talking about hiking for two plus hours.

You must pay attention to 3 things: inner core temperature, hydration, and cardio.

You must check your inner core temperature. We now know that you should not exceed 101 degree F for your inner core temperature. While you are hiking -- about 20-25 minutes into the hike -- stop and using the rectal thermometer, take your temperature. If it lingers under 100 degrees F -- you are okay but know that your core temperature is beginning to rise. Because your babies do not have any way to sweat and regulate their own body heat, they could potentially get too hot.

Many women have made the mistake of thinking they could gage how hot they were by how much they are sweating. As you know, you could be hiking along on a cool day, not sweating too much but your body is really working on the steep inclines. This activity may spike your inner core temperature.

With each and every workout, I want you to begin a journal. Not only will this be a cool thing for your child to have later on in his or her life but this will help you analyze your own workouts over time. After each hiking or cardio workout, I want you to record the day, time, weather, how you felt, what you did. I want you to make note of what you ate for breakfast and prior/during the hike, what you drank and even what you wore.

What I'm wearing??

Yes. Different fabrics, even a hat determines how differently your body breathes. Finally, write how you feel after the workout. Tired? Energized? Blue? Whatever it is, write it down. We will be able to see a pattern that will help you have better, safer workouts and learn the pattern of hormonal surges.

Stay hydrated. Given what you do ... I am sure you are well aware of the powers of water. Still, here I go. The typical lecture is that most American women are naturally dehydrated and don't even know it. Drinking more water will help with morning sickness, water retention and, better for muscles development, circulation, and energy.

There seems to be the on-going debate on whether a woman can or should drink caffeine while pregnant. This is an absurd debate as we know the answer. While the cola and coffee industries are busily finding studies to offer health benefits to caffeine -- there are none for the pregnant woman and little for anyone else. You do not need to be naturally dehydrated by the caffeine and you certainly do not need to deal with anymore headaches. If you are a heavy caffeine drinker -- let's wean you slowly but let's get you off. Again, this should be part of your journal. Write what you drink. Over time, you can take a look at this to see how -- if at all -- you are progressing.

Finally, use common sense. As a seasoned athlete, you know what is best.

4. Horseback Riding, Scuba, Skiing, and Water Sports

Only weeks pregnant, my husband and I went skiing. I'm no skier so there was no danger of me crashing headlong into a tree because that would actually require speed on my part. Baby bunnies perched atop the bunny slopes snickered at me. I was S-L-O-W. When I did fall – twice – it was a pathetic, slow motion, fall-to-the-side kind of a fall. No snow was harmed in my embarrassing flop. But on the second slow-mo fall, my husband stopped to help me. I looked up just in time to see a large something headed like a freight train right for Robb. I could only open my mouth before the other skier slammed into Robb, spinning him violently some ten feet down the hill. Robb is a big guy and a very good skier. Even still, it was remarkable that he was able to stay on his feet. Had that been me ... I shutter to think. And that's the point.

157

I offer no false pretenses about my athletic abilities on skis. I have none. But even safely tucked away from the other skiers – I thought – danger lurks.

Over the years, I've answered questions and fielded comments from recreational athletes, weekend warriors, and seasoned veterans on the slopes and in the saddle about their love of horses, skis, snow mobiles, jet skis, surfing and the ocean. I've also conversed with multiple Olympic, national, and professional athletes in these sports who happened to be or were once pregnant while training. The irony is the women who were professional athletes, who most lived for their sports and could least afford to take time off were the ones who always scaled back their routines. Because they understand the risks involved.

There is a long-standing joke in the world of martial arts. Black belts do NOT like to spar green and purple belts (who are new to the art of sparring). While strength is important, the art of sparring has much more to do with skill, balance, strategy, and control. Green belts get excited when they spar and tend to whoop-up on whoever they are fighting, moving in like giant windmills. The inexperienced fighter is the most dangerous – not the black belt.

Now that you are pregnant, there is no wave, no ride, no ocean, no horse, no mountain worth hurting your baby for. That said, let's take a look at some different scenarios:

Question:
Aloha! I am a little over four months pregnant and still surf shoulder high waves with grace. When should I discontinue, or can I carry through until the end? I can't imagine a week passing without catching waves. This has been my life for over five years. Some advice would be much appreciated. Mahalo.

Answer:
There are some conditions you must factor in...

In terms of physical activity, it is always difficult to answer such questions without knowing the history of the person.

You Must be given permission to continue with physical activity from your doctor -- meaning there are no medical reasons or conditions that should keep you from such activities.

This should be an activity that you are already conditioned to do. After five years, I would say you have acclimated to the demands of surfing.

And you must stay hydrated. You know better than anyone how dehydrating it can be working out in salt water, in the sun, using all your muscles for balance/poise on the board, staying hydrated is critical.

Therefore, take more breaks, monitor how much water you drink. Given all this -- again, be sure that you are a seasoned surfer and that your doctor. is on board (figuratively), go for it!! As your body changes -- affecting balance -- you will naturally move away from the board until the baby is born. But have fun now while you can.

But we have to factor in the danger element! We often discourage women who are pregnant from skiing and cycling outdoors because of one major factor -- other people. The most seasoned skiers and cyclists have to contend with first time skiers on the slopes, careening out of control or motorists not paying attention or dogs attacking. These outside factors MUST be considered as a matter of safety for mother and baby. In your case, there are some things you just cannot control -- the waves, other surfers. Please consider these factors as you enter the water.

Question:
"Hello! I am 5 weeks pregnant and this weekend I went water skiing. The nurse at my OB/GYN said it was fine for me to go although she said this was to be the last time. While water skiing I feel face first (like a belly flop) into the water one time very hard. I've been concerned ever since. Could this have hurt the baby? I'm feeling fine and have no pain that us unusual but I'm just the worrying type."

Answer:
It's good that this was your last time, thus removing the temptation to try again. While I've had clients who water-skied into their fourth month, this is one of the sports I tend to shy away from because of the outside factors -- like belly flopping. It's unlikely that your untimely belly flop did any real harm to the baby. But I'm sure it's been frightening all the same.

I advise women how to train well into their eighth month but have a short list of no-no sports. Cycling (outside), skiing (both water and snow), scuba, horseback riding, motorcycling, 4-wheelers ... any of the sports where water/waves/snow/other cars or competitors can crash into you should be avoided.

The fact that you have no pain and no bleeding would indicate that all is well. Still, play it safe and schedule an appointment with your OB/GYN for your own peace of mind. My advice: no worries but hang up your water skies for now.

"Horseback exercise carried to fatigue seems occasionally to have conducted to pregnancy."
                                    -The Physical Life of Woman, 1872

[Interestingly, while they once again have it backwards, this may be one of the first early observations that the "active" woman is healthier, thereby in better constitution for conception.]

159

Question:

"Can you tell me if it is safe to go horse riding when you are eight weeks pregnant. I am not a regular rider, in fact, I haven't been on a horse for years but have recently been asked to go and agreed before I knew I was pregnant."

Answer*:*

Do not go. This is absolutely not the time to saddle up and go. Even if you were an avid rider, I would caution you against going but a greenhorn has no business riding while pregnant.

I know you agreed to go before you knew you were pregnant but no friend would want you to go and risk hurting you/the baby. Take a rain check.

Question:

"I just recently found out that I'm pregnant. My family has been planning a Christmas vacation to Colorado to go skiing. Can I ski? I will be about nine weeks pregnant. I'm a very cautious skier on blues. Could I do easy green slopes or it is too dangerous? Do you have to fall hard to miscarry? We usually ski twice a year for a week. I have been running the past eight months about 12 miles a week and doing aerobics for the last two years."

Answer:

Nope, nope, nope. My skiing little friend, if you have read any of my material, you may know that I am a firm believer in the power of the pregnant momma. I trained for the US bobsled team while pregnant. However, I never got IN the bobsled to slide on ice. There are several no-no's in sports for pregnant athletes/moms. Scuba, horseback riding and skiing are tops on the list. Scuba is obvious and in a class by itself but many moms argue they are in condition for horseback riding and/or skiing. These sports have outside factors -- like bobsledding -- that have nothing to do with your level of athleticism. May I remind you of the two very high-profile skiing accidents with the Kennedy family and Sen. Sonny Bono. Both were accomplished skiers -- both lost control on the slopes and were killed. In the case of a weekend-warrior skier with plans on staying on the bunny slopes, you are still in great risk of being plowed over by novice skiers. If you were cross-country skiing, I would be more enthusiastic. As long as you remain properly hydrated and do not get too hot while skiing, this is a safe, reasonable exercise. As for skiing on the slopes, the risk is just too great.

I know this is disappointing news to you and I applaud you for being in excellent condition (Keep it up!) but steer clear of the slopes. Again, the risk is too great and will not be worth it to you should something go awry.

Question:

"Hi, Alex. I will be 8 weeks along when I am planning on going on the whitewater kayaking trip of a lifetime! I am an avid kayaker (go twice a week for the past two years) and know my abilities are perfect for this trip. Should I be concerned? Also, what is the recommendation for wakeboarding?"

Answer:

Okay, I would say given your athletic/kayaking background, you certainly do know your limitations and abilities. First, let me lay out my worries and you can wade through them, decide what applies and/or how to make proper adjustments for your upcoming trip:

In regards to the kayaking:

-- Proper hydration: You know better than anyone that it is very easy to become dehydrated while kayaking. Oh, the irony of being surrounded by water and slowly dehydrating. But this sport can be long and demanding work, not allowing time for water breaks. You need to be sure that you take these breaks for proper hydration and to allow your body to cool.

--Inner Core temperature: I know, I know... you're in a kayak. You can't exactly leap out and take your inner core temperature. Therefore, weather is more important than ever. Be sure you do not overheat. You can demand that you set the pace for your group so that you can properly monitor how hard you are working and allow your body to sufficiently recover. This would mean keeping a check on your heart rate.

--Get medical permission. It would seem that you are in excellent health but I want to be safe and insist that you are cleared medically before launch.

--Whitewater. Ahh, now there is something to ponder. Just as I do not know your medical history, I don't know what class (rapids) you'll be riding. In smooth water -- no worries. But with rapids, anything can happen, even to a seasoned athlete. I was once asked to test drive a Gravity Car for Volvo. The test drive itself was super fun and easily within my abilities ... that is, until one of the brake systems snapped and a truck went around our barricade and came dangerously close to running me over! No one could have foreseen these potential disasters! I know this seems like an opportunity of a lifetime for you but the really important issue here is your baby. I do not question your abilities but worry about outside factors you cannot control.

Finally, the wakeboarding. I'm sorry to say that as much as I love wakeboarding and believe that you/baby would be fine after doing a number of good runs, we just can't know about those outside factors -- crashes, wiping out from a passing boats' wake, things in the water ... you get the idea. There are just too many unknown factors. For these reasons, it is better to be safe than sorry.

Question:

"I am 5 months pregnant with a normal pregnancy. No complications. I was wondering if it is safe to ride snowmobile? Is so, how careful must I be about riding?"

Answer:

As with horseback riding, cycling (on the streets) and skiing, the actual activity is riding the snowmobile is relatively safe for you at 5 months. This assumes you are not performing stunts and flying over bumps, putting your body through more of an impact-oriented activity. But like horseback riding, cycling and skiing, doctors do not recommend this activity -- not because they are concerned about your physical abilities/endurance level but because of outside factors you cannot control. The best skiers, for example, are blindsided by an inexperienced skier. Horses spook, cars run cyclists off the road. The dangers of hitting something hidden beneath a blanket of snow, a tree or another snowmobile are too great.

Add to this a rough course and it could indeed be far too much bouncing for the fetus. Not enough studies have been done on rough-terrain endurance and welfare for both pregnant momma and the baby. And really, who wants to risk being the guinea pig?

I hate to put a damper on such a fun outdoor activity but for the welfare of you and your baby, consider another winter sport. Cross-country skiing is a great, safe activity.

Question:

"My husband and I are going on vacation to a lake. We go water skiing and tubing. I will have ovulated a couple of days before we leave. Can I hurt anything by skiing or tubing if I am only a couple days pregnant? I just don't want to do anything to hurt my baby. Thanks."

Answer:

Boy, these questions are always tough to answer. We're working on some 'ifs' here. The truth is, if you are pregnant (days/weeks) your baby is the size of a rice. He or she is incredibly insulated and protected. The biggest dangers are dehydration and overheating. Having said this, however, there are some exercises that experts shy away from: scuba diving is the biggest no-no! Following scuba diving is horseback riding, skiing, water skiing, and cycling. It's been argued by many that "I've never had an accident!" or "I'm a great rider!" but outside factors such as a log in the water, a careless mistake by the boat driver, a freak wave, or even a slip on your part can create an accident that you can't control. I advise that you avoid high-speed skiing or tubing if you believe you might be pregnant. I am sorry to say this but it really is better to be safe than sorry.

Question:

"I just found out I'm pregnant but we planned a trip to Idaho. We were planning on going snowmobiling and I'll be about 7 weeks. Is this ok?"

Answer:

These are always tough questions. Here's why...

Physically, the activity of snowmobiling ... the bouncing, the impact of hitting slopes, the cardio exercise (hanging on, hooting and hollering!) are all fine – for you. But what of the baby? While your baby is well insulated, it's still a gamble how much of the rough ride might be too much for the fetus.

The other problem is the accident factor. I do not like activities such as horseback riding, cycling (outside), skiing, waterskiing, snowmobiling, to name a few, where you cannot control the environment. By this I mean, when you train in a spinning class, your bike is stationed. There is no chance of a rogue biker smashing into you. But in these other activities, you could lose control and hit a tree, get hit by another vehicle, crash or worse. While it's easy to say this won't happen ... it could. So, this question is less to do with "can I do this physically" and more to do with, "should I take the chance." Only you can decide. My personal recommendation would be 'no.'

Question:

"My husband and I planned a trip to Colorado pre-pregnancy. Now I'm pregnant and will be about 4 weeks when we take our trip. I am an expert skier. Is it too much of a risk – or can I still ski? Take it easy? Please say 'yes.'"

Answer:

Whoo, boy. I hate these kinds of questions.

I could talk to you about staying hydrated, watching your inner core temperature (please see information about inner core temperature or I will be happy to talk to you about it. Short version: Don't let your inner core temp rise about 101 degree F as your baby is one degree Celsius higher than your own temperature and has no ability to sweat). As an expert skier, this tells me that you are well-conditioned, have excellent muscle memory and should be able to handle the exercise without exerting yourself beyond a reasonable level. All good.

As an expert skier, I would also assume that you are in good medical health -- although you still must see your personal physician and/or OB/GYN to get medical permission to continue your physical activities and exercise routine.

Let's assume that you have excellent health and get the green light from your doctors to exercise. Now.... comes the tough part.

Experts typically do not condone certain activities such as skiing because expert or novice, there are outside factors you cannot control. There are all kinds of unexpected and uncontrolled situations which can cause you great bodily harm. *sigh

So, here is my response. In terms of the exercise itself -- you should be fine. As long as you stay hydrated and not allow yourself to get too hot, you should be fine. It's just the fact that someone could smash into you or cause you to veer off course into a tree or another skier. With this in mind, you should talk to your family, husband, doctor and make your decision.

Question:

"My girlfriend is nine weeks pregnant and we were wondering if it was safe for her to kayak, and if so, is it safe for the rest of the pregnancy? This is not whitewater, just a slow moving flat river. Almost no chance of tipping and no rapids. I know I would have to carry her boat for her as lifting the 50 lbs, is out of the question. This would not be new to her as she kayaked a lot before we found out. Any help would be great."

Answer:

Well, I would say you guys should be able to go kayaking -- but let's put out a few guidelines. The good news is that she has done this before and there are no rapids.

I always tell my clients that the sports/activities that have 'outside' risk factors have to go. For example, horseback riding (where you can thrown), scuba, snow or water skiing (where you can seriously wipe out or get smashed into), cycling (chased by a dog, run off the road ...) ... should be avoided. Recently, I was asked about surfing by a semi-pro surfer and pretty much said that while she was acclimated to the sport, was in great condition and certainly had the skills to continue, the risk of getting slammed by a wave or hit by a reckless greenhorn surfer was too great.

In the case of your girlfriend, she's got several things going for her. This is not a new sport and she is most likely acclimated to the sport. Most often, physicians will tell a pregnant athlete to stop because of any undue stress to the body. This is old thinking. We now know that as long as the body/muscles are acclimated to an activity, there is no stress. You will be doing the heavy lifting (but truly, if she is conditioned to carrying the kayaks, she can continue this into her second trimester), and there are no outside factors like crashing rapids or flipping.

My main concerns here are 1) she discusses this with her OB'GYN anyway. Because I don't know her medical history, I can't know if there are other medical conditions that I should be factoring in. 2) Heat. I don't know where you are kayaking but heat needs to be considered with pregnant women. Simply put, the baby has no sweating mechanism and has no way of cooling him/herself. As your girlfriends inner core temperature spikes, the baby gets hotter and hotter and there is evidence to support that there is a danger of exceeding 101 degrees F. Read up on how to use the rectal thermometer to safely gauge her heat index.

Along with staying fully hydrated, this is your safest measure for momma and baby. Again, the good news is that she should be able to stay fairly cool with your planned activity but be safe. Have a rectal thermometer and plenty of water on hand. Be sure you have the doctors' thumbs up before you launch.

5. Basketball, Bowling, Soccer, Volleyball, Softball, Golf, and Tennis

"Tennis is such violent exercise that one cannot recommend women to make use of it, except with a good deal of caution. Golf has the advantage of keeping its votaries much in the open air, without greatly fatiguing them. Some of the postures are very ugly, it must be confessed. The woman golfer may find it necessary to stand with her feet apart when addressing the ball, but she should be careful not to do so away from the links. It is an extremely ugly and unfeminine attitude."
                                                                    -Social Customs, 1911

Question:
"I've been playing tennis competitively for years. I am almost two months pregnant and feel pretty good, except for the morning sickness. Can I keep on playing safely?"

Answer:
Once you've spoken to your doctor and OB/GYN and have been given permission to proceed, you should be able to continue with some qualifiers.

Whether you are playing indoors or out, you must pay attention to your inner core temperature. This may be more difficult during a match so you need to speak with coaches, teammates, and opponents about this prior to practices and matches. I don't know the level of your competition but you have one main priority right now and it must be the baby. Be sure not to exhaust yourself or become overheated.

Stay hydrated and check your inner core temperature.

That said, you must also be aware of your changing body. At two months, you are indeed strong. But as your body changes – ligaments soften, joints shift – you may be more susceptible to injury. Tennis, like basketball, demands side-to-side moves that may put undue stress on your knees and hips so pay attention to your body. Listen to and respect those changes.

Because very little study has been done on pregnant tennis players, you have to rely on your own judgment. Tripping, twisting too deeply, and charging/falling into the net are risks. Perhaps you will need to consider playing half-court or doubles.

Most athletes stop when the sport is no longer fun or feels go. To protect your knees and hips, you will most likely gravitate toward stationary cycling, Stairmaster, or treadmill-like exercises.

Question:
"I play netball (basketball) once and sometimes twice a week and have done so for a long time. But now I am pregnant and don't know if I should be playing. Can I still play at all and, if so, when should I stop playing and find another form of exercise?"

Answer:
The good news is ... you are acclimated to this kind of exercise. But, before you play another game, you need to speak to your personal physician. Because we do not know what your medical history is, you need to get a clearance from him or her. Be sure to explain to your doctor that you also want to keep playing basketball. Our biggest problem -- and this is why most doctors do caution pregnant women away from cardio sports (sports that make you run and sweat) – is women get pregnant and decide they want to work out. This is NOT the time to decide to get into shape. But it sounds like you are already used to the sport. This means your body is adjusted and should have no troubles
continuing the sport. Assuming that your doctor tells you that you may continue with the sport, there are factors to consider. Heat index. While you work out, your inner core
temperature will rise. As icky as this sounds, you will want to purchase a rectal thermometer. Your baby's body temp is one degree Celsius higher than yours. And your baby has no sweating mechanism so, as your inner core temp rises, so will the baby's. For this reason, you want to be sure that your temp does not rise above 101 degree F. So, while you are playing, you can dash off to the bathrooms and take your temp. I know, I know ... but Olympians and professionals do this while pregnant to ensure the utmost safety for their baby while working out/training.

Also, be sure to stay hydrated. As much as we hear experts tell women to stay hydrated, the vast majority of women are dehydrated and do not even know it. Stay away from colas and coffee. Drink plenty of water and, yes, it will seem like you are going to the bathroom all the time but this is just another way to be sure your body stays cool and hydrated for baby.

Now, as your pregnancy continues, your belly will expand. As your grow, you will most likely back off from more aggressive games of basketball. But we want to warn you about twisting ankles and knees. Particularly with sports such as basketball, this can be a problem. As your pregnancy progresses, your joints will loosen and ligaments will soften, possibly putting stress on your hips, knees, and lower back. I would caution against aggressive ball playing by the middle of your second trimester. While your baby is well insulated, you need to protect YOU as well. Basketball is not for the fainthearted and the competition can easily get heated -- I mean that in more ways than one.

Listen to your body. When you start to feel sluggish or slow... be respectful. You can continue to play but go for defense. Eventually, you will probably just want to ride a stationary bike and lift (light) weights to stay in shape. Please keep us posted as you move along but, again, get that rectal thermometer and talk to your doctor.

Question:

"How long can I continue to play basketball? I think I got pregnant about a month ago. I don't play too physically. I play with my husband, brother, and other guys at the gym in pickup games. How long can I continue to do this without hurting the baby?"

Answer:

It sounds like you are already in good shape and conditioned for basketball. This is an important point. We typically tell women who are pregnant that they may continue with their physical activity as long as they are conditioned for that particular sport/movement. Too many women get pregnant and THEN decide to get in shape. Again, this is not the case with you so, I would say that you can continue to play but we have a few "howevers."

You must get permission from your physician. I do not know what your medical history is so it is important that you let your dr. know what you are doing. Be sure to tell Team Baby how intense the pick-up games get. About the pickup games -- stay hydrated. Believe it or not, most Americans are dehydrated and don't even know it. Yes, you are going to be going to the bathroom more than ever as it is but I must still insist that you drink a lot of water. How do you know you're doing a good job?? Your urine should be almost clear. The darker it is, the more dehydrated you are.

It is very easy to overheat. Many moms-to-be will ask, "Yes, but won't I know how hot I am?" Not necessarily. Your inner core temperature should not exceed 101 degree F -- because your baby is one degree Celsius higher than your own temp and your baby has no sweating mechanism, you have to be sure your temp doesn't suddenly spike. This is easily caused by activities that include sprinting/sudden bursts of energy -- like basketball. So, how do you know what your inner core temperature is?? Ah, so glad you asked.

A rectal thermometer.

So, you're drinking water, staying hydrated, not overheating. You are playing with family who will undoubtedly look after you. My only other concern -- again, this all hinges on the green light from your doctor -- is hitting a wet spot or sweat spot while you're on the floor. I am assuming you are on a wood floor. As your body changes, your joints do soften and you want to be sure you do not slip/slide. So, be cognizant of your ever changing body and eventually, you will decide to taper off from the boys. When this happens, contact me again and I will give you some hints/ workouts to stay in shape for the rest of your pregnancy. Meantime .. she shoots, she scores!!! Go for it.

Question:
"I suspect I am pregnant. Is it okay to continue playing golf this summer if I am? Is there any point at which I should put the clubs away? What about toting clubs? I am in moderate shape, though carrying a few extra pounds, and had no complications during my previous pregnancy."

Answer:
Okay, before I can say 'yes', you need to check with your OB/GYN and personal physician, as I do not know your medical history. I always want to be sure that there is not another medical factor that might cause problems.

So, assuming you are in good health and have permission from your doctor, there is no reason you cannot continue. We have a few rules, however. I see you live in Denver so I am not as concerned about heat. However, I suggest that you read about inner core temperature. We have information posted about this. Multiple studies have been conducted about strength, mother-fuel, nutrition and genetics but few athletes have been taught about what happens when your inner core temperature spikes as a result of prolonged workout. In short (and please read more about it), your baby has no way of regulating his or her own body heat and will heat up as your inner core temp spikes. Do not exceed 101 degrees F -- inner core temp. Learn how to monitor inner core temp by using a rectal thermometer.

The rule of thumb has been, continue doing whatever you are doing. I am always most concerned by women who get pregnant and THEN want to get active. But because your body is already acclimated to this activity, you are not putting any undue stress on yourself, heart, joints...   As you move along, you will feel how your stance and swing will inevitably change as a result of your growing body. One concern doctors have with pregnant athletes is deep twisting. Pay attention to your swing. While it will certainly alter your game a bit, you may want to modify the swing. Always listen to your body. As long as you are comfortable, as long as you feel strong -- you can continue. Most athletes -- even the weekend warriors -- gradually step away as it becomes "unnatural" feeling. At that point, stay active. Walk. Lift light weights. Keep your muscles active and strong.

Question:
"I'm a fairly small woman (5'2", 107 pounds), and not super fit. Almost the only exercise I do regularly is playing volleyball – once or twice a week. We play tournament style on an indoor court. I just found out I'm pregnant and wonder how long I can continue to play. Or, should I not play at all? If I were to pick up some exercise during pregnancy, what would you recommend?"

Answer:

You need to speak to your physician before you do anything else. Because we do not know your medical background (or any problems/complications you may have), we must be sure that your physician is aware of your activities or what you plan on doing and get the medical green light from him or her.

In regards to the volleyball (and assuming you are allowed to continue physical activity), there should not be a problem. You should be able to continue play as you have. Volleyball is seasonal so you have time to finish out the season and re-prioritize before a new season begins. Most likely, you will find that after this season (possibly a second) you will want to do a more structured, individual workout, i.e. cycling, Stairmaster with light weights.

Our biggest concern is when we have a newly pregnant person who suddenly decides to take up a new activity after becoming pregnant. But if you have been playing volleyball for a while, your muscles are acclimated to the moves and strains of the game. During your first trimester, we are most concerned about overheating and physical exertion attributed to heavy lifting. This is not a problem with your sport. Because you are in a temperature controlled environment, we simply ask that you stay hydrated and resist dives. (FYI: My eldest daughter now has a broken foot as a result of volleyball -- a stray ball came under foot as she was doing a jump/hit.)

Were we talking outside volleyball during the summer months, I would discuss inner core temperature with you. (Read more about inner core temperature and heart rate in Chapter 4).

By your second trimester, your body is changing/joints softening and intense volleyball may be too much. The good news is, this is not supposed to be a contact sport but as you read about my daughter, accidents happen. Again, this is when you may want to re-think your exercise routine.

So, let's say you decide to go for a more structured workout at the gym. The next obvious step is to talk to a personal trainer who has dealt with pregnant clients. You don't want anything wild or radically new. But you want to keep your muscles strong and lean (as much as your pregnancy will allow), maintain your cardio and stay strong. Think in these terms: come your labor and delivery, you want to be strong and cardiovascularly fit for the physical event of your life -- and that of your babies. We know that moms who work out while pregnant have better, easier, happier pregnancies and are apt to have easier deliveries and recover more quickly. Therefore, you want to find someone who can teach you proper form on weights (light weights, higher reps), using cardio machines/cycles and ideas for home workouts. Walking, for example, is an excellent way to stay in shape and keep your cardio up and legs strong. Even if you can only afford one session with a trainer, make the investment for a safer workout routine.

Question:
"Is it okay for my wife to bowl? She's six months pregnant."

Answer:
The easy answer is "yes." However, there are some conditions. As long as your wife was bowling before her pregnancy and this is an activity she is used to, by all means, bowl until it is no longer comfortable. The American Medical Association allows women to continue with low-impact activities throughout their pregnancies as long as this is not a new activity. Having said this, it is important to note that as your wife moves into her third trimester, her joints will begin to loosen -- the body's way of getting ready for childbirth. It is important that her upper body strength is such that she can easily handle (and throw) the weight of a bowling ball. Even the backwards swing of a ball that weighs too much can cause possible hip/knee/lower back injuries for your mother-to-be.

New moms often try to prove to everyone that they are fine and can easily handle weights they cannot. It isn't that they can't handle the weight but with their changing physique and loosening joints, something as light as a bowling ball can be cumbersome.

As a bowler, be sure to watch her stance and throwing arm to be sure she is comfortable at all times and, of course, be sure to get a clear bill of health from your OB/GYN before you let her slip on those bowling shoes!

Talk to your wife's OB/GYN and personal physician to be sure she is medically cleared to continue this activity. We need to be sure there are no other medical problems, including old back injuries, that might cause problems while bowling.

Question:
"I'm 40 years old and confirmed yesterday that I am pregnant. I had a miscarriage a few months ago. I am on a woman's bowling league and have been since last May. The league ends in April. Is it safe to continue to bowl even though I am a high risk? What about prenatal yoga?"

Answer:
You must contact your doctor and discuss your 'high-risk' pregnancy. That is the first thing you must do. Because we do not know all the details of your medical background and because you recently miscarried, it is difficult to answer this question based on such little information.

However, if 1) your physician is comfortable with your continued bowling and believes you are physically able to workout and 2) you have already been working out and your body is acclimated to elevated heart rates, cardio and other muscle regiments, you should have no difficulty working out.

If you have been working out regularly and bowling with consistency, there will be no 'shock' to your system. In fact, studies show that women do better during pregnancy when working out.

They recover more quickly and have easier deliveries but, again, this is all contingent on the fact that your body can handle the exercise.

Yoga? Again, once you are given the green light from your OB/GYN, yoga would be a nice way to stay in shape, stay loose and keep your muscles strong. But check out the yoga class. You don't want a hot house – or hard core routine that will put new stress on your body. Yoga can be quite strenuous.

You must first speak with your doctor, then employ a personal trainer who is certified and experienced in working with pregnant clients. [Broke? Even meeting with a trainer for a one-time-fee of $40 is money well spent for a safe workout routine and peace of mind].

Stay strong! Walk with hand weights, eat well and join a support group to keep you energized, educated and motivated throughout your pregnancy.

Question:
"I've enjoyed reading your articles on how pregnant women who have already been living active lifestyles can continue to be active throughout their pregnancies. I play soccer, and would have liked to continue to play it a little further into my pregnancy (I am 9 weeks gone), but the season is drawing to a close, saving me making the decision at all. I plan to start jogging twice a week, in place of soccer training, and I am encountering resistance when I discuss this with family and friends. I intend to mention this to my doctor at my next visit, but though I have had no complications, and this will be my second child (first pregnancy had no complications whatsoever), it is my experience that doctors always err on the side of caution, and I feel that I will probably be advised to 'take it easy', and try walking, or swimming. Please can you give me some ammunition so that I will be able to discuss this with my doctor in such a way that I can show that I have done my research, and encourage him to move away from his 'cautious' recommendations?

PS. I also cycle to and from work each day – approx 3 miles each way. It is mostly flat roads, with one hill on the way home. Do you have any thoughts on how long I should maintain this?"

Answer:
Firstly, congratulations on your pregnancy and being a very fit, healthy mom. It sounds as though you've made fitness a priority in your life -- undoubtedly which helps you remain a healthier and happier mom. In this regard, I can arm you with some bits of information to share with your friends/family and to discuss with your doctor.

Why run? Why not? If you are perfectly healthy, have been running during soccer and want to continue, why not? Understand that you will most likely decide at some point in the pregnancy to begin power walking in replace of running. I have known a number of women who ran throughout their entire pregnancy but these women are rare. Most women decide within the second or third trimester that it is no longer comfortable to run and move to walking. You can tell your doctor and family that you have a plan in regards to running:

You know that you need to make sure you are always hydrated. Many people think that by drinking 'some' water, they are hydrated. Not so. You need to be sure you are drinking throughout the day -- not just gulping water before a run. You will propose that you intend to cut out or down on the caffeine if you are a caffeine (coffee, cola, tea) drinker.

Before you run, you will check the weather and air quality. For safety reasons, you will run with a buddy.

You can educate them about your inner core temperature. Explain to them how you will job/walk with a rectal thermometer and will be checking your inner core temperature for the safety of the baby. Explain that your baby does not have a sweat mechanism which means his or her body temperature will also rise. For this reason, you do not want your inner core temp to rise above 101 degrees. This keeps your baby within a very safe and comfortable temperature. If you are running for one hour on a cool October day, I would not be worried. However, should a runner head out for a long, long run and become very hot, this is a problem. You would need to stop every 20 minutes -- ducking into a bathroom, behind a tree in the woods ... whoever you are ... and take you inner temperature.

Now, the long term benefits. You mentioned that you are lifting weights as well. Excellent. I recommend working with a trainer -- just once or twice -- to be sure that your weights and body positioning are proper when working out. As you move into the second and third trimester, meet with the trainer again to be sure you are moving/lifting/standing/pressing properly. Again, this will please your friends and family. You understand that as your body grows and ligaments shift (as they will), that you will need to adjust how you train with weights!

But cardio is also important. The weight lifting will keep your muscles strong and toned. But you will also need to work your cardio for the day of childbirth. I am always surprised by the number of people who are surprised how HARD labor is. Scientific studies have shown that women who worked the cardiovascular throughout their pregnancy had a faster, easier delivery and recovered more quickly! Because your endurance will be top notch, because you've kept your abdominal walls pliable, because your lower back and muscles are conditioned and because you have trained mentally (a runner's benefit), labor and delivery becomes more of a sporting event that you will better handle than a sedentary woman.

Moreover, when you train throughout your pregnancy, endorphins are released -- natural hormones that help keep you more optimistic, happier, and healthier -- you are more inclined to be aware of what you eat and drink. Whereas sedentary mothers-to-be put on more (fat) weight and have poorer diets. You will be less likely to experience postpartum depression and this is important to note as mothers are more apt to suffer from postpartum depression with baby #2.

Finally, you are running because you want to and you understand that when it becomes cumbersome, you can go to power walking with 1 or 2 lbs hand weights. Run for fun, run for comfort, run for you!

Question:
"I just started up another season of soccer and am five weeks pregnant. It's a recreational league. What are your thoughts?"

Answer:
Without knowing much of your background, let's lay some ground rules first. **If** you have been playing for some time and are already conditioned to the sport of indoor or recreational soccer and **if** your OB/GYN and primary physician have given you the green light (this is important because we don't know if you have other medical issues to be factored in) and **if** you feel strong... here are my thoughts. You go, girl!

But... ah, there are usually many buts involved. A few things must be considered and you must tell you coach so that you can be rotated frequently. Inner core temperature. This is an important topic. As your body heat spikes, your inner core temperature rises, leaving the baby no way to sweat. Your baby cannot sweat AND your baby's own body temperature is one degree Celsius hotter than your own. Therefore, you should not allow your body temperature to go above 101 degree F. So... you're wondering how will I know. The biggest mistakes athletes make is thinking, "Well, I'll know when I get really hot." Not so. Particularly in sports like kickboxing, soccer, basketball... where sprint work and sudden burst of energy are required. This spikes your inner core temperature and there is no way for you to know exactly how hot you are until you are officially beyond the point of safety.

1) Stay hydrated. Drink plenty of fluids throughout the day, not just during the sporting event.

2) Carry with you a rectal thermometer. I know, I know... you're thinking "icky" and your baby is thinking, "whew! she's going to find out how hot it is in here!!" Dash off behind the bleachers, in the trees, in the bathroom, in a car... wherever you can go to check your inner core temp. It's not very pleasant but it is the best way to ensure the safety of your baby. What's more important than that?? Within a one-hour event, you should check yourself at least twice.

3) Watch your sprints. You will frequently read that your heart rate should not go beyond 140 beats per minute. This is torture for women who are athletes. The reality is this. You may exceed 140 beats per minute, however, you may not stay above 150-160 beats per minute for prolonged periods of time. Translation: You can have your break away with the ball, run it down the field, shoot and score! Then, you need full recovery. As long as you allow yourself recovery time, you

should be fine. The danger is keeping your heart rate elevated for prolonged periods of time. Do not be afraid to raise your hand often, asking to be subbed out.

In the book, **Entering the Mother Zone** (which can be procured through www.pregnancy.org). The book profiles athletes from all walks of life, even US soccer stud Joy Fawcett, who talks about how they trained, what they did, ate, drank and recovered from sport. It's another great resource for the pregnant athlete.

Finally, let's talk about how physical the game of soccer can be. We can keep you hydrated, get you to carry and use a rectal thermometer, check your heart rate, heat index and overall strength. We can't estimate the jerk who is going to slam into you, knock you down and steal the ball. This must be your decision. Talk to your teammates and coach and ask them how they feel about you playing....

6. The Extreme Sports of Pole Vaulting, Rock Climbing, and Flying High

Question:
"Hello. I am currently 10 weeks pregnant and 19-years old. I have been pole vaulting for 14 years and am an All-America in the sport numerous times. Knowing the risks involved with pole vaulting there is potential to seriously get hurt if I miss the pit. Also, I am concerned about the fall onto the mats from such a great height. (I jump around 14 feet). Would this be way too dangerous to continue at this time, or would it be better to limit myself to drills where I land on my feet with a handhold about a foot higher than I can reach while standing with my arm extended? Should I even do this at all? Part of my problem is that I am coaching girls' pole vault and have to show them what I want rather than explain it."

Answer:
I understand your situation completely. During my third pregnancy, I was also a kickbox/karate instructor. When new students came in, I felt the need to demonstrate. Let's break this down point by point.

There are a number of risks involved with your sport. That is true. One of your biggest problems will be balance. As your body changes, this will throw off your technique in the way you carry and run with the pole, and vault. The good news is, you're in great shape. Cardiovascular speaking, you should have no problems. Because of your muscular conditioning and muscle memory (that is, your body knows what to do/how to move), you'd be amazed how well your pregnant body accepts continued physical activity. If you were running, cycling, even a competitive fencer, I'd say, "no problems." But because you are using a pole and vaulting to great heights, this is a concern. Here's what I suggest:

1) Talk to your OB/GYN. You MUST have medical clearance before you

continue. I don't know your entire medical history, so you must rely on your physician's expertise.

2) Assuming you are indeed in good health, be sure to stay properly hydrated and check your inner core temperature should you work up a good sweat. Please review our information on inner core temperature. Unfortunately, few trainers and physicians seem to know (and advise) on this topic. In short, it is a way to be sure that you do not exceed an inner temperature of 101 degrees F. Your baby is one degree Celsius higher than your own inner temperature and has no way of sweating. By checking your inner core temp, you can insure that your baby will not overheat.

3) Skip the pole, limiting yourself to drills where you do land on your feet. Even then, we will have to modify this as time goes on. But for now, your muscle memory is such (again, assuming that you are good to go medically speaking) that you can do this activity. Pregnant athletes report that they knew when it was time to back off even more. If you have a funny feeling or question about what you are doing, my advice is always "back off." You will be back in top form in no time. Remember, that given your age, you will bounce right back!! Don't worry.

4) Get yourself an able bodied assistant. This is great for a number of reasons. This really will sharpen your skills as an instructor/coach when you explain the movements and then have someone demonstrate. You can stand there and break down what and how your assistant did what she or he did. This will really help your young athletes as well. But by using an assistant, when you really CAN'T jump anymore, you will have a seasoned assistant and someone who can step in for you when you are out.

5) Don't sweat it. People understand pregnancy. You will be pleased by how understanding and supportive the moms will be. You've got a great resume and will be just as effective instructing rather than demonstrating.

Question:
"Are amusement park rides safe during the first trimester?"

Answer:
Yikes!

If you've read my e-mail responses about surfing, horseback riding, rock climbing, running/jogging, soccer, swimming .... as so on .. about sports or other thrilling forms of physical activity, my response is typically "yes" IF 1) you have your doctor's permission (as we do not know your medical history), 2) this is an activity you are conditioned to, 3) you watch your inner core temperature (not applied to amusement park rides), and 4) you stay hydrated.

With sports where outside factors, such as getting hit by a car (cycling), thrown from a horse, and smashed into by another person (skiing, surfing) I am more cautious. But with amusement park rides, there is far too little information known to say this is a safe activity. You can't "condition" yourself for amusement rides. You're just a body flailing in a seat!

To compound this, there was the terrible story of the healthy 11-year-old boy who died on a roller coaster ride at Disney World in 2006. The fact is, the G-forces on many of today's amusements rides are anywhere from 3 to 5 G's -- translation: the equivalent to what fighter jet pilots train for in their jets. I'm sorry to say but fun or no fun, it's too risky. Sit it out and ride the easier water rides!

Question:
"I have been indoor rock climbing for several years. Is it safe to continue during my pregnancy if I limit myself to top roping?"

Answer:
As you are already experienced in the sport of rock climbing you/your body is acclimated to the physical demands. Good for you. The general rule of thumb for pregnant athletes is you may continue your activity until you feel the need to let up. Obviously, scuba is out! And sports where you cannot control outside elements -- other skiers, cars, cyclists, horses -- are discouraged. I asked the Allen family (Tori Allen is 3xWorld Rock Climbing Champion) about harness/safety belts are was told competitive climbers stop free climbing after the first trimester and resume wall climbing. Again, only until you feel discomfort should you stop. However, you must realize that this is a sport of balance -- something you may struggle with as your body grows.

Be sure to consult your physician, including him/her on your regiment. If you have further questions, bring your safety gear to your next appointment to show how it fits your body. In the meantime, climb and enjoy.

Question:
"Is it safe to participate in indoor rock climbing? Can the intense stretching needed to pull my body from rock to rock cause the fetus to detach?"

Answer:
Because this is a relatively new sport in regards to studies on pregnant athletes, there is very little data on the training regiments, stretching techniques and injury statistics. Therefore, I have a few questions. Is this a sport you have been participating in for some time and would call yourself a seasoned climber? This is important because your body must be acclimated to the kind of pulls, lifts, stretches required of such an incredibly strenuous sport. Is your doctor fully aware of this activity and has s/he given you the medical green light to continue? Are you wearing all the protective gear and training with a trainer?

If the answer to all these questions is 'yes', you should be able to continue but you must listen to your body. As your body begins to change/expand and the weight shifts, it will affect the way you climb, thereby changing your reach. As the pregnancy progresses, concentrate more on technique. Take your time and, as they say, enjoy the scenery -- yes, even indoors. You will reach a point where you decide to ground yourself and begin working light weights, perhaps pre-natal yoga to stay limber and strong.

Question:

"I have a question, having just discovered my wife is pregnant: Is it safe to fly during the first 12 weeks of pregnancy? She is supposed to fly from Europe to the United States for a business trip next week and I have heard people say this is unadvisable. What would you advise?"

Answer:

Yes, she may fly until her third trimester. Even then a pregnant woman can fly but under the advisement of her doctor, as each case is different.

However, the flight from Europe to stateside is a long one. She will need to get up once every 45 minutes or so and walk around. Even a trip to the ladies room will help her stretch out her legs and get the blood flow going.

I also highly recommend that she drink lots of fluids -- specifically water. No colas. No coffee. As the cabin pressure changes in the airplane, it also affects our bodies. I'm sure you've heard that air is "recycled" and that is why so many people get sick on airplanes. The truth is most people are dehydrated BEFORE they step onto a plane. The air and cabin pressure change only makes matters worse. Your wife can stay properly hydrated (and walk around a lot because a pregnant woman will certainly have to use the restroom more often when drinking more water), and fight common colds by drinking.

Question:

"I glide. Can I do this while I am pregnant? I am four months along and wanted to know how long I can do this? What about the altitude?"

Answer:

What about the altitude?!? What about the landing?

On a normal airline flight, there should be no problems with traveling. Typically, by the seventh month, OB/GYN's and personal physicians urge pregnant women to stop travel for long periods when they would be cooped up and avoid high altitudes. Circulation and blood flow are the biggest reasons for this.

But you are talking about something completely different. This 'extreme sport' kind of travel is not safe for you or the baby. The risks of crashing or even having a hard landing are too great. I would say your hand-gliding days should be over until after the baby is born.

7. Your Team/Your Journal

From bowling to basketball, soccer to rock climbing, the big questions are always "How much can I do?" Without your team, your options are limited. Each day you should be journaling your activities, how you felt, and what you did so that you can show your actions and results to your team.

Who is the team again? Your OB/GYN, personal physician, trainer, nutritionists, coaches, teammates, buddies, and family.

From time to time, a well-meaning team member may ask too many questions or, rather, appear to question too many things. Remember that they are concerned for both you and baby. Many times, it is easy to forget how often we push ourselves during pregnancy in the quest for one last repetition, one last shot, one final run . . . Team Baby is looking out for both of you so be open to suggestions, be willing to share your journal with your medical team, and don't forget why you are really working out.

Chapter Eleven
Your Ever Changing Tummy

Question:

"I just discovered yesterday for the first time that I'm pregnant but I have a concern. While opening a jar, I accidentally pressed it against my tummy. Is it okay? Will it affect anything? Also, before I knew I was pregnant, I was involved in some vigorous activities (i.e. company run and body combat) and I've not exercised for a while prior to that. Is it okay?"

<u>Answer:</u>

Hi! You made me smile with the jar pressed against your tummy question. I remember those days ... This is why I do what I do. During my first pregnancy, I did not know anything and each "first" was scary. I actually fell on my stomach late in one of my pregnancies. Talk about scary.

Peace of mind is a powerful thing so if your worries continue to plague you, ask to see the nurse at your OB/GYN just for a listen to your baby's heartbeat. That should make you feel so much better. In the meantime, however, I would not worry about the jar pressing against your stomach or company run and combat training. (Although I do hope you write back because I am so curious about what it is you are doing. Military? Reserves? I would love to know.)

My biggest concerns would be if you had become dehydrated and how hot your body temperature was. Having said that, at 4 weeks, you would be AMAZED how resilient your baby is. But I want you to do a few things.

1. Talk to a trainer about becoming more active. I say this because you will find that women who worked out during their pregnancies have an easier time during labor and delivery. Not only are your muscles stronger and able to endure a long labor (most inactive women are reportedly very tired and sore), but you will also rebound more quickly, have more energy and heal faster. Women who work out regularly during pregnancy are more likely to feel better and happier, less likely to become depressed, less likely to keep on the baby weight gain, and are -- overall -- healthier. When you do this, you are more likely to eat more healthily.

2. Focus more on water, shy from the caffeine.

3. Learn more about inner core temperature. When you read [Chapter 4: What Your Trainer Isn't Telling You] and understand what inner core temperature is and how to get the temperature accurately -- this will give you tremendous peace of mind.

Regarding the jar business... do not worry. You are about to have plenty of 'firsts' but as you do, you will quickly learn that as your body changes you will bump into things and your body is more than equipped to handle it. There are plenty of stories of women who fell from or trip over something, women who have run marathons, hauled farm equipment during their entire pregnancy. (Uh, not that I'm suggesting marathons or farm equipment).

The last piece of advice is this: women always ask how they will know when they should lay off of oh, say, aerobics or lifting boxes. While there are scores of time frames -- some say do not lift heavy objects once you've entered the second trimester, for example -- the one thing all experts agree on is "listen to your own body." If it doesn't feel good, don't do it. It's that simple. Because women are built so differently, because we all have different levels of conditioning, of pain tolerance, and of strength, we simply can't give a guideline. Listening to your own body, how you feel, is your best defense for healthy living.

1. Abdominal Exercises: What Can I Do?

Of everything that is going on, you are most aware of your stomach. Of course you are. What both physicians and trainers want to see, however, is a positive awareness of your expanding belly. This is not the time to be thinking about "burning fat," "trimming the tummy," or "keeping the six pack." There will be plenty of time for that later, after the baby is born.

Often, when I am asked the question, *"Can I do sit ups?"* I respond with a question of my own. "Why?"

There is sometimes a pause. "Why why?" We are at an abdominal impasse. They wonder why I would wonder such a thing and I must wonder what the objective is for performing crunches or sit-ups.

Question:
"Is it okay to do sit-ups or crunches during the first few weeks of pregnancy?"

Answer:
The answer is somewhat controversial. You will find some studies that urge women to stay away from abdominal exercises in the first trimester, others that suggest you stop after the second trimester (allowing for the first trimester), and others still that suggest nothing at all for fear of detaching the fetus from the uterus wall. What's a mom-to-be to do?

But before I answer this, I want you to consider why you want to continue abdominal exercises. If you are under some grand delusion that you might be able to decrease your girth, stop excess belly fat, or somehow create a more svelt prego-mid-section by doing crunches, let me help you out. Allow for this time to be one in which you focus on what and how you eat, sleep, and drink. Focus more on your upper body and legs rather than how large your middle is becoming. Trust that your body knows what it needs to do and that you are busily creating a beautiful new baby.

That said, I would hope that if you want to work your core it is simply because you understand that a strong core will help eliminate lower back aches and will enable you to do better in the labor and delivery room. A strong core will, in fact, help you recover more quickly after the baby is born. For these reasons, I would applaud your interest in abdominal exercises.

The easy answer is that if you are in good medical condition, if you have already been exercising, and if you have medical permission, you may continue crunches. I recommend crunches of the ball. (see Part III: abdominal exercises).

Avoid lying flat on your back. Instead, choose a decline board or my personal favorite, the ball.

On the floor, you may lie on your side, performing side crunches. In fact, I did the side crunches throughout my pregnancy. No jerking, no tugging – but slight, gentle crunch ups on each side.

If you have never exercised before or are new to crunches, this is not the time to start alone. Contact a trainer and (after you have been given medical clearance) work together on a safe, gentle program that will allow you to build better core strength.

Question:

"Is it okay to do full sit-ups while I'm pregnant? I have to do these to pass a test at work but want to make sure it's okay and I won't hurt my baby."

Answer:

Let's assume you have medical clearance and are in excellent condition. Let's also assume that you've been doing sit-ups for some time and are acclimated to this exercise routine. Finally, let's continue the assumptions in that you will not be jerking upward, trying to do something like 50 sit-ups in 60 seconds but that you have a minimal amount you must do and thus, will be able to do controlled, smooth sit ups. Whew! These would be the only conditions that I would feel comfortable telling someone they could continue doing sit-ups in the first trimester.

If you have not been given permission to do this, are not fully acclimated to this exercise, or are expected to perform a high number in a timed event, I would not do this.

Because I do not have all the information on your personal and medical background or what kind of physical test this is, I would advise that you meet with a trainer. Let him or her know what is expected of you and let the professional assess your present condition.

I know this is for your job but safety should be your main concern.

Question:
"I have the 6-Second Abs for Crunches, in which you sit in an upright position. I was wondering if that would be safer than traditional sit ups and crunches while pregnant?"

Answer:
Of course, this is contingent of several things... You must first get permission from your doctor. We do not know your medical history so we want to be sure that you have been given medical permission to exercise. Assuming that you have, we must also consider how far along you are in the pregnancy. The main reason physicians and trainers ask that pregnant women NOT lie on their backs while exercising is for both mom and baby. The pressure and weight of the baby can make oxygen flow more difficult so it has always been suggested that women remain upright. The reality is this -- do what is comfortable.

For my own clients, I allow them to continue full crunches into the beginning of their second trimester but we focus working on the ball, avoiding a flat back on the floor. While doing crunches, do not jerk on the back of your neck if you clasp your fingers behind your head. Instead, interlace your fingers in front of your chest, gently putting your thumbs under your chin. Each time you do a crunch, lift your chin as though you are trying to touch your chin to the ceiling.

By your third trimester, you can perform side crunches (with or without weights) on either side, still working the obliques but not putting undue strain on your lower back or the baby's oxygen supply. Even on the ball, some women still report feeling like their air supply is limited while crunching. If this happens to you, the side crunch (on a mat) is the perfect solution.

Still, my favorite workout for abs and pregnant people is with the ball. The ball -- be sure to get the large exercise ball -- will absorb much of the pressure your lower back and hips would otherwise absorb on the floor. Sitting on the ball, you can roll forward so that the ball is centered in the small of your back and, with hand weights, you can do several variations of crunches. It's great for your breathing, the baby, low-impact crunches and isolating the stomach muscles for a nice workout. How can you be sure of what you are doing? You can find several exercise ball workout guides at Barnes&Noble or on-line. My favorite is the **Swiss Ball: For Strength, Tone, and Posture** by Maureen Flett. Fabulous!! Good luck and keep on crunching.

The research on pregnant women who worked out throughout their pregnancy -- particularly ab work -- show faster labor and delivery, speedier recoveries, better overall experience while pregnant and happier/healthier disposition!! You can crunch but use common sense. Remember, this is not an exercise for a toned stomach but rather an exercise to ensure a better/easier time in the delivery room.

Question:

"I read on a previous question that after the first trimester floor crunches are not safe because it lowers your blood pressure and is dangerous. Does this rule apply to bench press and other weight training exercises performed on a bench or floor? What about incline bench? Also, does this mean I can't sleep on my back after the first trimester? This is my first pregnancy but I have been weight lifting (moderately) and running my whole life. Very concerned."

Answer:

To be clear, dangerous is not quite the right word for someone who is accustomed to exercise and, specifically, crunches. The problem is, there is no absolute so why risk it? Using common sense is your greatest weapon. Many years ago, I had a fellow instructor perform abdominal crunches where the legs are thrown down to the ground. She was seven months pregnant. It was no surprise to many of us -- who tried to stop her but she wouldn't listen -- that some scary complications followed. The end result of that story is ... you can work out but you can't be stupid about it.

I continued to do crunches through my pregnancy -- even the day before -- but I was always careful. I took my time and perfected nice, slow lifts. Here's the low-down:

Before I say anything more, I have to ask that you talk to your personal physician and OB/GYN. Because I don't know your medical history, there may be extenuating circumstances I are not aware of. Explain to the doctor what your previous exercise routine has been, the kind of condition you are in now and how you plan to work out. But if they tell you not to work out based on medical conditions, listen to your doctor(s).

Having said this, it sounds like you are in a very good position. Because you already workout, you already have muscles/tissue that are acclimated to exercise. What always worries me is when I have a new client who is quite sedentary, gets pregnant and suddenly wants to get in shape. Yikes. But because you work out regularly, because you have a routine and your body is already in tuned with these demands/movements/strains, you should fare well. So, don't get crazy and try new things at this point. Stick with what you know/what you like. This does include crunches.

At 9 weeks -- I know you know this -- your babe is an itty bitty rice. Ahhh, but a beautiful rice and one that cannot regulate heat. Therefore, you need to be sure to:

1) stay hydrated

2) do not overheat. You can take your inner core temperature (I know it sounds dreadful but it's the best way to be sure you and baby are safe) by using a rectal thermometer. Here's why: You cannot "tell" how hot you really are. Clients ask, "But can't I tell by how much I'm sweating?" No. Your baby is one degree Celsius hotter than you -- at all times. As you work out, your body temperature spikes. Right when you think you're feeling pretty good, your inner core temp could spike

without you even realizing it. You want to be sure that you do not exceed 101 degree F. Thus, the rectal thermometer. After about 20 minutes of a running/cycling/aerobics routine, dash off the bathroom and check your temp. This makes sure you stay in the safe zone.

3) Get a journal and begin marking your workouts, how much you do, how you felt after. It is even better if you can mark your dietary patterns. I don't care about weight gain -- and neither should you -- but by marking down what and how you eat, you can see a pattern of when (or if) you get fatigued more quickly, feel dehydrated or get too hot too fast. Many times, my clients will believe they are properly hydrated. Then, we look back at what they ate and how much they drank water ... surprise! Not enough.

4) Continue the moderate weight lifting but as you move into the second trimester, work with a trainer. Even if you can't afford a trainer, do it just two or three times. You want to do this because your body is changing and without realizing it, your position will change to accommodate the changing body.

Be sure your trainer has worked with pregnant clients before. Again, you should do this in the beginning and end of the third trimester. Again, it is a safety precaution.

We snicker and giggle about this but many of us get "hormonal" while pregnant. In truth, a natural hormone is released while pregnant that can act as a steroid. Some of my clients who are already athletes or gym rats will become suddenly Xena, Warrior Princess on me. I'll walk up, tap them on the shoulder and ask, "What do you think you're doing?" By periodically checking in with a trainer, we can keep the Xena out of you -- for now.

5) Crunches. Again, my main concern is inner core temp. As long as you are not straining, you may continue with crunches on the back – but why not use the ball. This "no-back" rule is really designed for women who do prolonged and heavy activities on their back but it's always better to be safe. It is more of a precaution than anything else. You are perfectly able to safely do crunches in the first trimester. Experts maintain that this can continue into the second trimester.

Finally, on sleeping. You may sleep on your back in the first trimester. However, most women report that they feel more comfortable on their sides. Some women even sleep on their stomachs -- can't imagine that myself -- but again, it's safe. On this, the position of medical professionals is the same -- do what feels good. By the middle of your second trimester, however, it is "suggested" that you sleep on your side. I suggest investing in a body pillow. It is great while your hips are changing/expanding, it will help you sleep more easily

Question:
"I'm going on my second child and I haven't gotten rid of my stomach from my first (son). I'm wondering if there's any exercises I can do while I'm pregnant and after to make my stomach smaller?"

Answer:

In a word -- no. I'm sorry to give disappointing news but this is not the time you should worry about reducing tummy size. This is a very common concern among moms and the good news is -- there are plenty of things you can after the baby is born. Right now, to do exercises specifically geared to your abs or reducing calories is both futile and harmful to the baby.

Now, you can do moderate exercise and watch your junk food/soda/sodium intake to keep your body from gaining TOO much weight during pregnancy. I have worked with women who came out of a pregnancy the same weight (and in a few cases a few pounds lighter) they were before. It is important that you 1) talk to your OB/GYN about this and 2) get a referral to a certified nutritionist who has worked with pregnant women before. Together you can work out a great diet plan that will leave you energized, healthy, and full!

Beyond that, enjoy your pregnancy. Focus on having a healthy baby and we'll talk again after baby is born for working away your mommy tummy!

2. Oh, No! Something Bumped My Baby

Over the years, I've received countless letters and questions regarding a bumped tummy. From falling while water skiing to tripping down football stadium bleachers, the questions are posed in the same manner. Momma is fine but has a horrible feeling something has happened to the baby.

If this should happen to you, call and make an appointment with your OB/GYN. Even if you are not due for another appointment any time soon, do not allow yourself to be put off by an unconcerned or uncaring receptionist. Calmly and politely explain that you've had an accident and that you can't sleep until you know everything is okay.

 Why this advice?

 There have been very few times I've feared something might be wrong. Most often, a mom-to-be fell and banged her tummy with no further repercussions than a good scare. But why lose sleep over worry? Ask to be seen, go in and talk to your OB/GYN. Listen to the heartbeat for further reassurances. Given your concerns, your OB/GYN should not put you off.

In the end, you will sleep better.

3. Something Feels Funny

Questions:
"Am I supposed to be feeling anything on my tummy during the first trimester? Would I feel the baby's heartbeat by now? I am a bit worried since I am on my 8th week and as of yet I don't feel anything. Please advise."

Answer:
This is an exciting time! And more than anything, new moms want reassurances that baby is okay and thriving. Unfortunately, it is rare (very) for moms to really feel anything in the early weeks of pregnancy. Yes, eight weeks is considered "early weeks." Typically, you will feel other things first -- a heaviness feeling or actual expanding waistline, heavier breasts, or nausea. Do not panic. This does not mean you will continue to expand but, typically, the thinner you are, the more change you feel in the early stages. Conversely, the larger you are, the less change you will feel. Many women report having headaches, feeling tired or listless, and slightly nauseous. Again, all normal. Into the 2nd trimester, you may begin to feel activity from the baby.
Flutter feelings, almost as though you are having gas, are common symptoms.

When you have these kinds of questions, it's always a great idea to make a list and talk to your physician. Be sure that everything is okay, you are medically cleared so that you may begin some kind of exercise routine. Women who work out during pregnancy have healthier babies, easier pregnancies, quicker deliveries, faster recoveries and overall, better moods. But there is something else that few publications (let alone doctors)
talk about. When you work out, you are in better tune with your body. When you are in better tune, you will better identify feelings of your baby moving around. Fitness buffs who are also pregnant swear that they can even feel 'the mood' of the baby. The baby typically gets more quiet as momma works out and becomes active when momma is resting. It is a fun sensation, let me tell you.

But first thing is first .... get to your OB/GYN and talk about your medical history, the pregnancy and be sure you can work out. Meantime, just know that you SHOULD NOT worry about not feeling anything right now.

Question:
"I am about 10 weeks pregnant and lately I've noticed that when I stretch I feel a sharp "pulling" pain in my lower abdomen/uterus area. Is this normal? Should I be worried about this?"

Answer:
Often times, as your body changes (ligaments and joints), you may suddenly become aware of certain "pulls" in your lower torso. HOWEVER, let's be safe and

have you see your OB/GYN. It's a precaution, to be sure, but because I don't know your medical background and physical conditioning, we just want to be sure these are more common strains as your body changes.

You are wise to be proactive. I would much rather someone "pester" their doctor than wait only to learn something is really wrong.

Some women never experience any kind of pull or strain sensation, let alone gain more than 20 lbs during their pregnancy. But the rest of us gain more and feel more as our bodies change. Some women feel the change most often in the last trimester while others feel the biggest changes in the first trimester. The wondrous, mysterious thing about pregnancy is .... everyone is different. Because of this, it's always best to check things out. Your OB/GYN should measure your abdomen, make record of the changes/growth and discuss your physical activities.

Question:
"I am about 6 weeks along and my abdomen is tender to the touch. Is this normal?"

Answer:
It is not unusual for you to experience tenderness. However, we always suggest that you make an appointment with your OB/GYN. Most likely, you'll be told this is normal as your body is already changing and you will experience tenderness, sometimes a pulling/tightness sensation as your ligaments, joints, even skin stretches and shifts. But we want to be sure that everything is fine so .... make that call for peace of mind and safety for your baby.

Question:
"I'm currently 7 weeks pregnant. Ever since the pregnancy started, I haven't had much energy to work and I've rapidly gained weight in the belly. I'm wondering if it's the pregnancy or if I'm bloated. Is it normal to already have a belly at two months? What can I do to workout if I'm too exhausted?"

Answer:
Well, this is not at all uncommon. The frustrating part is we hear so much about women who have that glow or are ecstatically happy about being pregnant or have 'energy to burn' that it's hard to imagine the other and far more realistic side to being pregnant. Yep -- it can really poop you out! So, feeling exhausted and perhaps a bit disappointed, we should take this one step at a time. There are things you can and should be doing to help relieve these common symptoms.

1) Talk to your OB/GYN. Be sure to stress that you are far more exhausted than normal. I say this because it is very common for a patient to tell her doctor she's tired but get blown off. Unhealthy Americans as a whole are reporting feelings of

exhaustion. It's important that your doctor understand that this is something new for you.

Additionally, many new moms-to-be are anemic. Most women can go through their entire lives and be anemic without really knowing it. Except, when she gets pregnant. Total fatigue sets in and it can get to the point where you become dizzy, even disoriented. Make your doctor understand exactly how tired you are.

2) Pre-natals. A lot of women complain that the pre-natals make them nauseous so they don't take them. Your baby will take what he or she needs from your body (assuming that you are well nourished) but this can leave you feeling run-down. The pre-natals will help you maintain your energy levels while giving the baby what you need. Take your pre-natals. And, if they make your tummy upset, take them just before going to bed. This is a great idea for most minerals and vitamins as most are water soluble which means you flush out a lot each time you go the bathroom. By taking vitamins before sleeping, the thought is, there is better absorption of vitamins and minerals into your system. Most importantly, you sleep through what might have otherwise made you feel gassy or uneasy.

3) You are what you drink!

Remember these words. We have all kinds of evidence that shows drinking coffee or tea, for example, is okay. Therefore, we naturally assume that drinking soda pop and Gatorades are okay as well. The truth is, water is best. You should not be drinking caffeine and certainly do not need sugary drinks. This is added sodium and calories NOT needed. [Re-read Chapter Three: You Are What You Drink]

The sodium increases chances of weight gain -- particularly in the middle for pregnant women -- and morning sickness (or fatigue). Water, water, water.

Ah, you say... but then I have to go the bathroom all day.

Alas, it's true. But by drinking water throughout the day you will help decrease morning sickness, control your weight AND appetite, as well as help skin (as hormones change, break outs can be more likely), headaches and energy level.

4) You are what you eat. I hate to say it but we know that preservatives cause or can certainly trigger migraines, headaches, and low energy. Skip the fast food. I know that in today's busy, I'll-Super-Size-that kind of a world we live in, it's very hard to skip fast food restaurants but your baby, your waistline, energy level and body will thank you for it. Eating natural foods help the pregnant body do what it does best -- grow a healthy baby while maintaining a strong core. While your sweet tooth might be tempted, you can eat plenty of healthy, sweet (natural) things. Skip the high-fat frappachinos, brownies, and lasagnas!

Now, let's take another realistic look at two more things. Some women get pregnant and seem to grow a basketball under their shirts, not really putting on weight anywhere else. Unfortunately, that is what we typically see on t.v. But, guess what? More women than not gain weight. Period. You gain, you grow, and you know that when the baby is born, you can work to take it off. The two dumbest things you can do while pregnant is 1) diet or 2) decide you're eating for two. You are eating for you -- so choose wisely because now you have a baby taking what he or she needs from you so eating junk food is foolish. You will gain weight and that's okay!! But you can help dictate and determine HOW MUCH you gain.

The second thing is exercise. You mentioned you're too tired to work out. This pleases me because I know you are thinking about exercise. So, let's have a goal. Go back through the list of 1-4. Make that happen. Once you've begun this process, you will have more energy -- even if it's just a little. Step on that treadmill and go for a walk. Each time, add a little more to it. Finally, because we do not know your medical background, you need to be sure that you have medical clearance to work out. If so, talk to a trainer in your area. It doesn't have to be expensive. In fact, you can meet with this person just ONE TIME to be sure you have the proper technique, workout and body position. This is a safety precaution for you and baby. Once you know what you are doing, begin exercising and this, I promise, will give renewed energy.

Just remember that it typically takes about two to four weeks of exercise before you feel that you are getting more energy but it will come!

Chapter Twelve:
Your Ever Changing Mood and Appetite

No, you're not losing your mind. You may feel weepy one moment and overwhelmingly blissful the next. You're forgetting things yet can't seem to get the image of a big, fat, greasy burger out of your head. What's going on??

Psst. You're pregnant. But this is not a free-pass to throw temper tantrums or devour the All-You-Can-Eat diner out of business. Your moods do affect your baby.

1. I Forgot ... What Was I Doing?

If ever you needed a reason to get motivated about exercise, this is the one. Exercise helps you stay focused, keeps you more organized, set better goals, and complete tasks. This is important as your brain does actually shrink during pregnancy. A 1997 British study conducted by researchers at the Royal Postgraduate Medical School found there is evidence of "impaired cognitive functioning," causing loss of short-term memory and lack of concentration. But a new study about pregnancy and brain shrinkage may prove otherwise and, as you will read, much of it is connected to breastfeeding. Neuroscientist researchers at the University of Richmond and Randolph Macon College in Virginia conducted a study on laboratory animals to better understand the effects of higher levels of hormones during the childbearing months. The study found that a pregnant animal's behavior is altered because of a change in the brain – a change that occurs when brain cell structures called dendrites actually doubled. This is significant as the dendrites are necessary for communication between neurons. Glial cells in the brain, which act as communication conductors, also doubled, making pregnant mice more energetic, more aggressive, and more curious. And what were their rewards? Exercise. While they worked wheels and mazes, their energy levels increased. While you're no mouse ... this is all the more reason to exercise. Cheese, anyone?

2. I Want to Change My Eating Habits ... But I Can't!

You can. After my son's third visit to the emergency room in four weeks, it was clear that he was in critical distress. In January, 2006, we met with one of the leading pulmonary experts in children's pediatrics and he told me two things I already knew: my son was very sick and that something would have to change. Diagnosed with environmental asthma, it's pretty hard to dictate the wind and, in the state of Texas, even harder to regulate chemicals. So, we made two major changes in our life. We began an aggressive medical treatment plan (one that required two-hour breathing treatments around the clock) and we quit eating fast food. I thought the latter might actually destroy my middle child who would actively not eat at home just so that she could announce she was starving and would need to go through a drive-thru while we were out and about. Like most moms today, I'm busy. Three children equate to six soccer practices, three soccer games, one violin lesson, one guitar lesson, one horseback riding lesson, and two girl spirit meetings per week. In addition, I teach kickboxing and self-defense classes, write for the paper and am under a book contract. I am the fitness/nutrition expert for a non-profit pregnancy organization and do volunteer work. While I preach healthy living, I'd gotten sucked into the 'busy mom' syndrome and had justified eating on-the-run because "we had to."

Yeah, yeah, yeah… I know all the statistics on diabetes, trans fats, clogged arteries, childhood obesity, preservatives, and processed foods. Heck, I've conducted seminars on such topics. But none of that really affected my family, right?? I mean, we work out all the time and don't drink soda pop. So, we're good, right?

The reality fairy had to hit me right between the eyes. I was kidding myself and, in the long-run, hurting my kids. Katie, my middle one, had begun to think I had a money tree growing in my back yard. She had no sense of money when it came to eating out. She was actually learning to make bad choices with food and with every French fry, she ate less and less veggies. While I'm lucky that I have three naturally lean children, I am seeing more and more children with thick middles –a relatively new phenomenon in this country.

In turn, I was also making bad choices. By always allowing eating out to be an option, I didn't budget well with my time, money, or health choices.

As we left Medical City in Dallas, I made the announcement. No more fast food. I made one concession. We could get drinks while we were out. Because we live in a hot climate and I have such active kids, we were allowed to buy water, certain juices, and ice tea. I'd expected begging and pleading. I'd expected Katie to start foaming at the mouth whenever we passed a McDonalds. Instead, she never asked. Not once. No one seemed to miss that we stopped eating out. But the surprises kept coming.

We saved money. But most importantly, most surprisingly, most happily was the change in Tommy's health. While I cannot dismiss the importance of his new medical plan, his new health food plan was huge as well. It was everything I knew coming true before my very own eyes. Without the preservatives invading his body, his natural immune system was suddenly fighting back – and winning! And not so remarkably, my children's taste in food has fully developed – no longer coated by saturated fats, salts, and preservatives. Katie actually craves artichoke.

To that end, many visitors to the United States report instant weight gain because our foods are so saturated with preservatives, hydrated and partially hydrated-crap. Only when they return to their native lands are they able to lose weight again.

You really are what you eat.

Author Mireille Guiliano tells the similar tale: She came to America as an exchange student and went home fat. Preservatives, processed foods, grease, and American-sized portions nearly did her in. Tired of listening to Americans complain about their weight, she wrote the nationwide best seller, **French Women Don't Get Fat**, (Alfred Knopf, New York, 2005). Simply put, food that comes straight from the farm or the garden straight to the table is best. This would include buying organic eggs and free-range meats.

How we shop in grocery stores and what we decide to stock in our homes can make or break us. Here's a tip: Shop the outer perimeters of the grocery store first. This is where the fruits and vegetables, meats, and dairy products are.

Ten Practical Steps to Breaking the Fast-Food Habit

1. Make a Dinner Wish List with your children and set out to eat together as a family at least three nights a week.
2. Shop together so that your children can help make 'choices' with you while you discuss the different foods and health benefits. Get your children to think beyond taste.
3. Stop to smell the roses – or read the labels. The more you read, the more you learn. Together, you and your children will learn more about foods and flavors. Would you rather eat a popular ice cream with 56 ingredients you cannot pronounce or organic foods with a short, healthy, understandable list?
4. While shopping, visit the spice section and discuss what different spices do for meals. You will be surprised how much you learn about spices and seasonings while reading labels and talking about different meal plans.
5. Budget your travel time around after school or weekend events. If you know you won't make it home to prepare a meal, pack sandwiches, fruits, and healthy snacks in a cooler.
6. Get everyone on board with this plan! When everyone in the family agrees to the plan and is proud about making healthier discussions, it is far easier to break the fast-food habit.
7. Watch food portion. Use a measuring cup [1 cup] to dish out foods for adults and ¾ cups for children.
8. Drop the soda. Introduce milk, whole juices, and water, water, water. Sugary drinks trigger hunger signals in the brain, making you believe you want or need more food than you really do.
9. Exercise. When the kids are playing baseball or soccer, walk the fields. If they are in bed at night, pop in a workout DVD or simply do push-ups. Exercise decreases the need for junk food while sweat cleans out the toxins in your body.

10. Keep a food journal. Pick a day and begin documenting your meal plans, sit-down meals, and every landmark you and your family make in terms of health, fitness, and family togetherness!

3. I'm Happy, I'm Sad: Can My Baby Feel My Moods?

Yes. And all too often, women are embarrassed to discuss this with their doctors. This is what Team Baby is all about!! One out of ten women experience depression while pregnant. And while exercise offers a great buffer against depression, it's not a fix-all. If you feel unusually sad, be sure to talk to your doctor about this, write out your feelings in your journal and share.

Chronic or severe stress may have effect on the baby, according to researchers at Harvard Medical School. Marriage, money, work, and self-image can all be triggers but sometimes it's just good 'ol baby blues. Rather than dismiss the feelings as something that "will go away," talk to your friends and family about your feelings.

Stay away from people who love to tell those horrifying pregnancy stories. You know, "I was in labor for 87 hours and finally gave birth out my nose!"

Find things to laugh about. A recent study at Loma Linda University found that even thinking about something funny significantly boosts chemicals in your body that eases tension. These "feel good" hormones, beta-endorphins and human growth hormones, are believed to lower blood pressure and increase your immune system. So, have a good laugh!

"To have a beautiful baby, the mother should often have some painting or engraving representing cheerful and beautiful figures before her eyes, or often contemplate some graceful statue. She should avoid looking at or thinking of ugly people."

-The Physical Life of Woman, 1872

4. Making Love While Pregnant

Question:
"I am taking the opportunity to ask some questions for my newly first time pregnant wife. Is it okay if we continue love sessions while she is pregnant and what normal diet should she take even if she is in good health?"

Answer:
Congratulations on your first pregnancy. This is an exciting time, but also one filled with questions. It is extremely important that you consult with physician

(OB/GYN) to be sure she is healthy and comfortable. By comfortable, I mean that she is not nervous about harming the baby. Many first-time-moms become very anxious about making love for fear it will harm the baby in some way. Because she is anxious, this can make the love making process painful and/or uncomfortable. She needs to be reassured that the baby will not be harmed and it is perfectly natural for your love sessions to continue -- AS LONG AS SHE IS COMFORTABLE WITH IT. Be patient with her. You may find that she runs hot and cold. This is such a confusing, frightening, exciting and joyous time. Her hormones may make her very emotional. For her, love sessions may be best if you both snuggle and cuddle. Talk to her, ask to go with her to the next OB/GYN appointment and let her know you want what is best for her.

As for her diet, a well-balanced meal is best. Even if she were not pregnant, I would urge this. Today, too many people are trying to cut out important food groups (example, carbohydrates) in hopes of losing weight. Our bodies are machines that need to be properly fueled by all the food groups represented in the food pyramid. As a pregnant person, she needs to focus on smaller, more frequent, healthful meals throughout the day. Reassure her that she should not worry about how much weight she gains. Some women put on just a few pounds where others really pack it on. As long as she eats well-balanced meals, avoids junk foods and sugary drinks (soda pop, sweet fruit-like drinks) and does a moderate amount of exercise (walking, swimming...) she will lose the baby fat much easier after the baby is born. Talk to your doctor about her diet today and see what improvements need to be made. Have her keep a journal of what she eats for a week and let a nutritionist look at it. Remember, she will most likely be experiencing morning sickness soon enough which means she will have aversions to certain foods. For a brief period, she may not feel like eating at all -- all the more reason to make sure she has a balanced meal. The baby will take what he/she needs from the mother, leaving your wife tired and exhausted. Urge her to eat frequent (smaller) meals to give her energy, improve her mood and keep her immune system strong against common colds and flu.

Lastly, you can be most helpful by making lifestyle changes with her. Offer to walk with her and change your eating habits as well. It's no fun to eat healthy if the guy next to you is eating fudge brownies!

Question:
"My husband is making me feel guilty. He doesn't mean to but he keeps trying for us to make love and it is not something I want to do. Is this normal? When I wanted to get pregnant, I wanted to have sex all the time but now that I have my baby, it doesn't feel right."

Answer:

The key here is that you need to feel comfortable about having sex. You need to explain to your husband that your feelings are very normal and that you can't be pressured into anything. During the first trimester, it is very common for women to lose their sex drive somewhat. Between morning sickness and the excitement of being a "momma," pregnant women feel more obligated than anything else to have sex.

During the second trimester, otherwise known as the honeymoon period of pregnancy, feelings of anxiety, nervousness, and nausea subside and pregnant women show more interest in lovemaking. Still, this needs to be something you want!

There are mixed reviews on the last trimester. Some women report feeling sexually aroused while many more simply feel too large, awkward, and clumsy for sex. For many women, the baby has become an actual person and the idea of having sex is upsetting.

It's funny … so many couples take all kinds of prenatal classes but do not give time to their own marriage. While this is a beautiful and exciting time, it is also an anxious time filled with questions and new problems. Sit down and have a heart-to-heart with your feelings about lovemaking and any pressures you are feeling.

If these feelings persist, talk to your OB/GYN about this issue. Believe me, s/he has heard it all before and may have some excellent solutions for the two of you.

Chapter 13
Your Ever Changing Boobs

Aside from exercise and diet, most mothers (or mothers-to-be) have a lot of questions about breast-feeding. Some women love it and wouldn't do anything else. Other don't relish the idea of being at the beck and call of their baby at all hours of the day and night, but wouldn't think of reverting to infant formula. Whatever you do, whatever you decide, there is one undeniable fact – your breasts are changing.

1. The Support Team – Your Bra

As discussed in the first chapter, it is very important that you wear an athletic bra while you exercise. But this is not enough. You should also be sure that your day-to-day bra offers extra support as well. For now, it's best to shelve the pretty, delicate bras. Contrary to popular believe, breastfeeding does not change the shape of your breasts. This occurs right now while you are pregnant.

It's long been held that the fluctuation of milk, the lactating and releasing while breastfeeding is responsible for breasts sagging and, in some cases, getting smaller. But the tissue damage and shape of the breast actually occurs during your pregnancy. According to researchers at the University of California at Davis, breasts look smaller once the baby is born not because of breastfeeding but because as you lose weight from breastfeeding, you also lose fat tissue in the breasts.

What you wear now is important for the support of your breasts and back. And, according to some, getting an adequate amount of protein and vitamin C will also help the connective tissues in your body to build or maintain better elasticity with your breasts.

2. How to Work the Upper Boy for Support

Ahhh, another reason to work out. You may find, as many do, that as your breast size increases, you experience back spasms. The natural pull (weight of your breasts) causes you to stoop slightly, putting undue pressure on your upper back and trapezoids. Overtime, this can be quite painful.

Whether you work out at home or in the gym, you can do simple exercises to help relieve the stress and strain.

From lateral pull-down, shoulder shrugs, and one-armed rows to push-ups (see Part III), you can create better upper body strength and create a better body posture – all good for the breasts.

3. Breastfeeding and What It Means for Your Baby Down the Road

The idea here is to get you thinking about breastfeeding. That said, it may be entirely possible that you will simply not have enough milk or the baby may not latch on. This is a discussion to be had with a lactation expert once your baby is born. But let me put a few thoughts in your head as you prepare for your baby.

Right now, you are doing everything right for yourself – exercise, hydration, better nutrition, self-esteem, and attitude.

- Breastfed babies of two weeks benefit from the nutrient- and antibody-rich early milk called colostrom.
- At four months, a breastfed baby is offered better immunity to fight off allergies and asthma later in life.
- Nursing for nine months gives the baby all the essential nutrients needed for his or her developing brain. In fact, breast milk contains a fatty acid crucial for the baby's brain and muscle development which is not found in any formulas on the market.
- Children who are breastfed do better in schools, score higher on standardized reading and math tests, and have higher IQs.
- It is far less expensive and more convenient as milk is always ready and at the perfect temperature.
- Babies who are breastfed have less food allergies later in life and … the best yet, according to researchers at the University of London, breastfeeding is believed to be a small protective against obesity later in life.

4. Today's Attitudes: Our Growing Crisis

Man has a far less exquisite tenderness for his off-spring than woman. There is little else than moral sympathy which attaches the father to the infant. Paternal love does not exist save as a thing of growth, of education.
- *Sexology, 1904*

As much information and education we provide for mothers-to-be, little is made of the importance of breastfeeding until the baby has arrived. This problem is compounded by breastfeeding myths and lack of support from significant others. Breastfeeding is not a mother issue but a family issue.

An Ohio State University study found that 75 percent of mothers say their husband's opinion greatly influenced their decision to nurse. As a result, a great number of women do not nurse.

Fathers who are knowledgeable about the health benefits of nursing to the baby tend to be more supportive, the study found, while those who discourage breastfeeding may fear separation from their partner or envy the special bond between mother and infant. Many of the unsupportive partners felt that the amount of time the mother was spending with the baby was taking away from the time the mother and father used to spend together, and it also took away from the time the father might spend with the baby.

No surprise, fathers who discouraged nursing may also mistakenly believe that infant formula is better for babies than breast milk or worry that breastfeeding will make a woman's breast less attractive.

With this lack of support and Victoria Secret commercials running (in the middle of day so our kids can see it!!), there is a great deal of stress on new mothers. Add to this the unspoken fact that the first few weeks can be challenging and painful. But once the new momma gets past the hard part – just getting started, letting their nipples get hard, getting down the nursing routine, adjusting sleep schedules – nursing is a wonderful experience.

And the good news is when mothers-to-be have included their husbands in the process, by having them on hand while nursing or even pumping breast milk and allowing the father to feed the baby, fathers do support breastfeeding. Truly, this is a family affair.

5. Breast Implants

As the trend grows for more and more women to get implants, there are some things that need to be considered. Unfortunately, this is not the time to be reading this if you've already had breast augmentation. Both physicians and pediatricians would like to see women get implants only after they are done having babies as implants are linked to lower milk volumes and autoimmune diseases in nursing babies. So, if you are a woman with implants, even if you aren't exhibiting any immune response symptoms, your baby might not be strong enough to ward off any side effects. These health risks are very good reason to use formulas if you have breast implants.

Chapter 14
The Great Pregnancy Myths:
From Hair Loss to Miscarriages, Falling Down
And Standing Tall … We Got It All!

Have your wife's breasts declined since you courted and married her? It is because her womb has declined and rebuilding it will rebuild them and nursing up her love will rebuild both womb and breast. Come, court her up again as you used to before marriage and, besides reddening up her now pale cheeks, lighting her now lagging motion, you will redevelop her shriveled breasts. Stay home of nights from your club rooms, billiard saloons and lodges to read or talk to her or escort her to parties, lectures, concerts and you'll get well paid every time you see her bust.

   -   *Creative and Sexual Science, 1876*

Question:
"I've read some places that you can sleep on your back and that it's only a myth not to. But I've read other places that you should never do exercises on your back. And I've read that you can do abdominal crunches. Which is it?"

Answer:
This is a jumble of fact and fiction. Here goes:

In the 1970s, there were a number of studies that found that while in labor flat on her back, the blood flow to the baby could be compromised. The vena cava, a major vessel beneath the uterus, can be compressed when the mother is flat on her back. As a result, women were heavily encouraged to be sitting up, walking or lying on their sides while in labor. In truth, the actual contractions (at their peak) are what reduce blood flow to the baby during labor, which is why hospital staff are careful to place the mother at a comfortable incline position, complete with the pesty but greatly needed fetal monitor.

Sleeping on your back is quite another story. For the healthy mom-to-be, there is no reason she cannot sleep on her back. If blood flow was compromised, you would feel light-headed and uncomfortable.

However, for moms-to-be who have medical issues such as hypertension or maternal kidney malfunction, for example, it is recommended that they sleep on their left sides. Having said all this, I found that I was more "comfortable" sleeping on my left side, convincing myself that safer was better. But this was a personal preference.

Question:

"I have heard that stretching for something high (such as stretching for something on a high shelf) is not a good thing to do while pregnant. Is that true?"

Answer:

There are several issues here. The myth is that you can tangle the umbilical cord around your baby's neck by stretching or raising your arms above your head. Approximately 25 percent of all babies are born with the cord around the neck, body, or legs. There is nothing the mother can do about this and when properly monitored – with today's incredible technology – the problem can be quickly rectified. Please do not spend time obsessing over this.

Reaching can be the problem. Let me explain. Reaching for something high increases the probability of losing your balance. For this reason, many physicians err on the side of caution and tell patients not to stretch too high. The stretching, however, can be very good for you in controlled exercise programs such as yoga. However -- and this is the big however -- only if you have already been in an exercise regimen of some kind.

If not, be sure to talk to your doctor about what you can/should do for exercise while pregnant.

*Personal story: in my infinite wisdom, I decided when I was 8 or 9 months pregnant that I couldn't stand looking at a spider web in the corner ceiling any longer. I got a broom and climbed onto the side of the couch, reaching out across the room to swipe the web. And, in a brilliant physical maneuver, forgot how huge my tummy way, lost my balance, fell off the couch and landed (partially) on my stomach. I was terrified as, for the rest of the evening, my baby did not move. I did not feel movement for almost 24 hours and, in a panic, called my doctor and asked to be seen. She was okay but BOY OH BOY did I beat myself up.

As your body changes, your balance, among other things, will be out of kilter. Always use caution. Talk to you doctor and find a great workout program that will keep you strong and healthy.

Question:

"This is regarding my wife. She is developing stretch marks during the first six weeks of pregnancy. Can you let me know what are the preventions to be taken and specifically any creams or lotions to be used?"

Answer:

Genetics play a huge part in this. I know, it's not something you want to hear but she needs to accept. As she puts on weight, the skin stretches and the connective tissues tear. This is how things work. Some women develop stretch marks early on, others not until the end of the pregnancy. Please reassure your wife that all women develop some variety of stretch marks so she does not need worry. In fact, supermodel Cindy Crawford and an increasing number of actresses are becoming more vocal about the fact that they, too, have stretch marks that are simply airbrushed out of photographs in the press/media. And we salute those actresses who have come forward with the truth!

Having said this, some experts do believe she can do some things that will be more helpful. Will they prevent stretch marks? No one knows -- but the belief is that they are helpful in prevention. Drinking water (staying hydrated -- skip the caffeine) and taking vitamin C helps cell renewal and skin elasticity. This will help fight stretch marks. And there are a number of products over-the-counter to help with stretch marks. One product I like in particular is an organic product so there are NO potentially harmful chemicals -- safe for your pregnant wife and baby. It is called: Earth Mama Angel Baby Body Butter. It is made by "Natural Woman". This is a great stretch mark oil she can use anywhere she feels stretch marks may be a problem. It is, however, expensive at $28 a bottle. Again, you may find all kinds of products over the counter -- including the popular vitamin E oils and lotions.

Question:
"I am at the first stage of pregnancy. I am of average height and wonder if it is unsafe to put on high heels (including platforms) during pregnancy? If yes, during which trimester? What kind of footwears do you recommend?"

Answer:
Ah, the war between high heels and sensible shoes rages on. High heels – or the principal of standing tall on the balls of your feet – poses no danger to your baby. However, two problems do arise with women who are pregnant and wearing heels. First, many woman report feeling clumsier. Although scientific research shows no medical reason for this and the debate continues whether women really are more prone to injury during pregnancy, the fact remains that many women say they feel clumsier. For this reason, my recommendation is an easy one: if you feel awkward or clumsy, stay away from high heels or platform shoes. In all likelihood, there is no danger for your baby but a strong chance you could sprain an ankle or worse. Second, as you move through the pregnancy, your joints begin to loosen in preparation of childbirth. For this reason, many experts suggest expectant mothers stay away from high heels because you could cause injury to yourself and theoretically your baby should you take a hard fall.

The most common complaint in regards to wearing high heels is the discomfort it brings to the lower back, which is already tender due to the changes occurring in your body.

While there is no medical reason against high heels, it is my feeling that it is always better to be safe than sorry. Flats, tennis/athletic shoes, and sandals (with ridged, rubberized soles that offer traction on slick surfaces) are always best.

*In the last trimester, dress for comfort rather than style. At this point, your feet are bearing the brunt of all your weight gain. Typically, women actually go up a half size in shoe wear as a result of pregnancy. Be sure to wear a shoe that offers support, such as running shoes, in care of your feet.

Question:
"I have to go to the bathroom all the time! Should I not drink so much water? It's even affecting my workouts. I have to leave my step class to go to the bathroom!"

Answer:
I have a theory. This is Mother Nature's way of getting you ready for taking care of a baby 24/7. The inconvenience of your potty breaks are actually diabolically strategized practice-runs to get you ready for all the times your baby will cry at the MOST inconvenient times.

But seriously, do not take this as a sign that you need to cut back on water. You may have to use the restroom 20 times a day yet still have chapped lips (a sure sign of dehydration). Because your expanding uterus is putting pressure on your bladder, you will have to use the bathroom more often. Case closed.

Question:
"My mom says you leak when you're pregnant and there's nothing you can do about it! Every time I sneeze, laugh, cough, or even stand up too fast, I leak. Is there any kind of exercise that will help this?"

Answer:
Absolutely. It's a workout of a different kind. Toning the pelvic floor muscles, which control the leakage, otherwise known as Kegel exercises, will offer you more control. A University of Michigan study revealed that women who experienced leakage problems were significantly diminished in both late pregnancy and postpartum after performing Kegel exercises.

How to do a Kegel? It's easy. Contract your pelvic-floor muscles as though you were going to the bathroom and then stopped the stream of urine by tightening those muscles. That's a Kegel. Now, hold for three full seconds. Release, repeat. Perform these repetitions twice a day for a total of five minutes.

Question:
"Will regular use of a tanning bed effect my chances of getting pregnant?"

Answer:
While there is no scientific correlation between tanning and conception, the American Medical Association along with the American College of Obstetricians

and Gynecologists and the American Board of Obstetrics and Gynecologists highly discourage this practice. Unclean tanning beds can be a breeding ground for germs and bacteria, not to mention the damage done to your skin. While this is presumably all news you have heard/read before, you are obviously thinking about motherhood. Now is the time to begin caring for yourself – long-term! Once you become pregnant, your OB/GYN will become very vocal about discouraging tanning. Try instant sprays or lotions if you must but begin thinking about overall health!

Question:
"I have confirmed my pregnancy and really, the site (www.pregnancy.org) has erased many of my myths and fears. My husband has a hereditary hair loss problem. Can I prevent this in my child by intake of green coconut milk? Actually, I am not living in a tropical area but I love to have nariyal pani/coconut milk. Is regular intake of coconut milk harmful during pregnancy? If not, can I look forward for some help on the prevention of the above problem of hair loss being transferred to my baby?"

Answer:
As you already mentioned, there are so many myths regarding pregnancy, child birth and babies. Your question about hereditary hair loss is just one of them. Unfortunately, the consumption of coconut milk is just another myth. Believe me, there would be millions and millions of pregnant women consuming coconut milk by the gallons if this were really true. The reality is, the gene pool is far more powerful than any kind of drink you could have. Remember this, just because your husband and his brothers may have hair loss, this does not always mean their children will have.

Focus on the more positive things about your husband and that you will have a happy, healthy baby. Good luck!! And, rather than drinking coconut milk, be sure to take prenatal vitamins and get a health check up with your doctor.

*In this case, the worried momma wrote back, asking about "the green or unripen coconut's water." Like many queries, it was clear that she wanted to know if it was safe to ingest, not wanting to hear of the "myth" associated with nariyal pani. The response was:

Answer:
Before answering, www.pregnancy.org consulted several OB/GYN specialists and fertility clinics in regards to research on this topic. Again, the answer appears to be the same. While there are several ancient Indian remedies that make claims of curing hair loss, science always comes back to the same results: genetics.

However, as one specialist put it, "But it can't hurt. It's important that the water be purified so no harmful bacteria is consumed. Other than that, if drinking the water makes her feel better, perhaps it will make for a happier, healthier pregnancy."

There you have it. Good luck.

As for our own personal opinion, you will have so many important decisions to make regarding the baby and will face so many important issues regarding health, developing muscles, speech patterns, social skills, education and general happiness, hair loss does not seem so important. Focus on the things our can do to develop a great human being and 'don't sweat the small stuff.'

Question:

"I must say that your site has helped me from being jittery to being oh, it's not going to be that bad after all, I'm 6 –7 weeks pregnant. I have read almost all the questions but could not find answer to some of mine: While sleeping I have a bad habit of tossing and turning or lying on my stomach. Is it bad for the baby? Secondly, I have to travel a six-hour flight when I will be seven months pregnant. Is it going to be harmful for the baby? What precautions can I take?"

Answer:

There are many myths about sleeping on a pregnant belly. The reality is ... comfort is the biggest issue. In the early stages of your pregnancy -- where you are now, sleeping on your belly is perfectly fine. However, I always tell me clients to "practice" sleeping on your side. As the time will come that you are not comfortable sleeping on your stomach and then it really isn't that good for either one of you as you are losing sleep, you want to be used to sleeping on your side.

You can find a pregnancy pillow (about five feet long) or even gather two and three pillows to create the same effect. Sleeping on your side -- left is best -- straddle the pillow(s) between your legs. As you get bigger and your hips shift/joints loosen, you will find that having a pillow to cushion between your legs, lift the leg to reduce strain on the hip -- you'll be happier and more comfortable. But for now, do not worry.

Flying at 7 months requires a conversation with your doctor. Here's why: there may be many circumstances we do not know about your medical history, such as blood pressure, weight, even previous injuries. For this reason, your personal OB/GYN must make this assessment. Typically, a perfectly healthy woman having a perfectly healthy pregnancy is allowed to fly but with caution. She is told she must be able to walk around during that six-hour flight, drink plenty of water and be sure to watch for swelling of hands and feet. Best course of action: stay in touch with your doctor and continue to remind him or her that you're to be taking a flight in your 7th month.

Question:
"I've heard that exercise can cause women to miscarry. I'm so worried about that. But I want to keep exercising. How big is the risk really?"

Answer:
*Please read Chapter 4 to revisit the information regarding inner core temperature, heart rate, working with a trainer, and talking to your doctor.

In the case of a healthy woman, research shows that women are better off with some form of exercise rather than not. In a study with the Columbia University School of Public Health in New York, in fact, it is believed women were less likely to miscarry as a result of their exercise regime.

But, clearly, there are some women who should avoid every during pregnancy. When with a history of early labors, hypertension, unusual bleeding, an incompetent cervix, or a history of chronic disease of the heart, lungs, thyroids, or blood vessels must speak with their doctors. They are most likely women who would be well advised not to exercise.

There will always be all kinds of myths, theories, worries, and secret family remedies connected to pregnancy. Most likely, we search for miracle solutions because the miracle of birth is just that. It is human nature to try and match a miracle for a miracle. In the end, you must approach your pregnancy in this manner. You have a great responsibility. All you can do is ALL that you can do. Eat right, stay hydrated and well rested, listen to your body, and enjoy this time in your life.

Good luck!

Glossary

Aerobic exercise Any activity in which a person's heart and lung must work harder, pumping blood throughout the body and sending oxygen to the muscles

Antibodies Proteins in the blood that fight against germs and build a defense against disease

Antioxidants A substance that prevents or stops oxidation; oxidation is the combination of a substance with oxygen

Artificial Man-made; not natural

Aspartame Artificial sugar; also known as Equal or Nutrasweet

Asthma A breathing disease involving wheezing, coughing, and difficulty in breathing

Blood circulation Movement of blood through the body's vessels, caused by the heart's pumping action

Caffeine Substance found naturally in coffee, tea, cola nuts, and cocoa that stimulates the central nervous system

Calcium A macromineral that helps build strong bones

Calories Units used to measure the energy value of food; that is, how much energy we are able to use from the food stored in our bodies

Carbohydrates the body's most important source of energy; nutrients that come mostly from plants; found in foods such as bread, rice, potatoes and sweet things, including natural foods such as fruits and vegetables

Cell The smallest unit of the body that can carry out the basic functions of life

Cholesterol   A type of fat that clogs blood vessels

Complex carbohydrates   Starchy carbohydrates that are digested slowly and
evenly for more sustained energy

Dairy   A place where milk, cream, and butter are stored and processed
(prepared for sale); Also known as dependency.

Dehydrated   Having lost too much water or body fluids so that bodily organs
begin to shut down

Dependency   A building detached from (standing away from) the main house used
To keep milk and butter cool. Also known as a dairy, this building
had thick walls under a big, overhanging roof to keep the cool air
inside. It had vents to allow hot air to escape.

Depravation   To be deprived, to be denied or prevented from having something

Diabetes   A serious disease that is the result of the body not making enough
insulin, a hormone that helps get glucose, or sugar, into the cells of the
body to be used for energy

Diet   What a person eats and drinks on a regular basis

Endorphins   A group of hormones with pain-killing and relaxing abilities that are
sent to the brain to make the exerciser feel better

Endurance   The ability to sustain a lengthy physical activity

Excrete   To eliminate or get rid of waste matter from the blood, tissues, and
organ

Extract   To be taken from

Fat   The body's major form of energy storage

Fiber   Also known as roughage; the main part of all plant tissue. Fiber is in
different whole foods such as grain, certain fruits and vegetables.
Your body cannot digest fiber but it is needed to keep your body's
system clear and able to get rid of waste (to have bowel movements)

Fibers   Long connective cells of muscle tissue

Fructose   A sugar found in fruits and honey; the sweetest natural sweetener

Glucose   A sugar (about half as sweet as normal sugar) found in many fruits, animal tissues and fluids. It is also the body's energy chemical. Blood glucose or blood sugar is the simple sugar your body obtains from foods you eat in an attempt to convert that sugar (glucose) to energy.

Glucose Intolerance A condition in which a person has an excess of glucose build up in the blood, or elevated blood sugar levels, somewhere between that of a normal, healthy person and that of a person with diabetes. This elevated blood sugar level should be monitored by a doctor because it could be a symptom of on-coming diabetes.

Heart Disease A disease of the heart that is the most common cause of death in The United States and is usually brought on by obesity, poor nutrition, and lack of exercise

Hemoglobin   A substance in red blood cells that transports oxygen

Hepatits   A disease in which the liver, an organ necessary for humans to live, becomes inflamed

Herb   A plant which has leaves, flowers, fruits, bark, or stem is used for medicine

Heredity   The passing of genetic factors, such as the color of hair or eyes, from one generation in a family to the next

High Blood Pressure Also known as hypertension; the thickening of the artery wall brought on by poor nutrition and lack of exercise

High Fructose Corn Syrup A chemically processed sweetener which interferes with the control of blood sugar and insulin resistance which raises the level of fat in the blood and causes your body to store more fat.

Hormones   Special chemicals a person' persons body makes to build muscle

Hyperactive   Unusually or abnormally active; this condition can be brought on by too much sugar and/or chemical imbalance.

Immune System Body system that creates a defense against foreign substances

Insulin   A hormone produced by the pancreas to help your body's cells use Glucose (or sugar) for energy. People who do not have enough insulin get diabetes, a disease which causes intense thirst, frequent need to urinate, blurred vision, and many more serious side effects, such as blindness and kidney failure (see Type II Diabetes), and requires daily medication.

Insulin Resistance A medical condition in which the body is unable to properly manage the insulin levels in the blood

Insulin Surges When too much insulin is released into the body, resulting in a rapid drop of blood sugar. This cause lethargy (extreme tiredness or fatigue) and sugar cravings, also known as hypoglycemia (a condition of low blood sugar)

Kidney Failure Failure of the kidneys; the organ that filters liquid waste from Your blood in the form of urine and helps regulate (keep watch over) the amount of sodium and water content in the body; failure can cause death

Lactic acid   A thick liquid that builds up in muscles during exercise, causing The muscles to be stiff and sore

Macrominerals Minerals needed by the body in large amounts; calcium, phosphorus, and magnesium

Macronutrients Nutrients needed by the body in large amounts; carbohydrates, fats, proteins, and water.

Metabolism   The process of how the body uses food to release energy and uses energy to build and repair body tissues; how your body burns fat

Microminerals Minerals needed by the body in small amounts; also called trace minerals; sodium, potassium, chloride, iron, zinc, iodine, copper, manganese, fluoride, chromium, selenium, molybdenum, arsenic, boron, nickel, and silicon

Micronutrients Nutrients needed by the body in small amounts; vitamins and minerals

Mineral   A material that is found in rocks and water and may also be found in our food. Minerals are important for a healthy body. (see macro- and micronutrients)

Monounsaturated (triglyceride) Unsaturated fats are considered the healthiest type of
fat, with none of the bad side effects that saturated fats have. Monounsaturated fats – such as olive oil, canola oil, peanut butter, and avocadoes – are thought to lower bad cholesterol (LDL) and reduce heart disease

Muscle A tissue made up of fibers capable of contracting and relaxing as the Body moves

Nutrients The material in food that your body needs to grow, create energy, and remain healthy/fight illness

Nutritious Nourishing, healthful

Obese A medical term for a person who weighs 40 percent or more than his or her ideal body weight. For example, a child who should weigh about 80 pounds but is obese actually weighs over 112 pounds – that means 40 percent more than he or she should weigh. Your doctor and parents/guardian should always work together to determine – based on your body structure and height – what your ideal weight should be.

Obesity Epidemic A term used to describe the spread of obesity (being fat) among people. Together, the Center for Disease Control and Prevention and the World Health Organization monitor how people around the world are gaining weight.

Obesity Rate The rate or number of overweight people in the nation and around the world

Organic Foods Food produced without the use of chemical pesticides and fertilizers

Organs Groups of tissue that perform specific jobs, such as the liver and gall bladder

Osteoporosis A medical condition in which calcium is lost from bones, causing the bones to become brittle and break

Overweight A measurement for weight; in medical terms, a child or adult who has 20 percent more weight (fat) than his/her ideal weight is considered overweight

Phosphates   One of the most common substances/nutrients in our environment, naturally occurring in our food, our water, and our bodies. The phosphate in soda pop is called phosphoric acid, and it adds tartness to the flavor

Phytonutrients   Foods that contain natural biochemical antibiotics. This is what gives fruits and vegetables their colors of blue, red, green, yellow, and orange

Polyunsaturated Fats   Like monounsaturated fats, these are the "good" types of fat, helping to prevent heart disease, lower blood pressure, and lover (bad) cholesterol. Polyunsaturated fats, found mostly in plants are soy beans, sunflower oil, safflower oil, corn, cottonseed.

Pores   Tiny openings on the skin's surface that allow sweat to come out and also let the skin breath

Protein   A group of chemical substances found in foods, such as milk and meat, that helps build our bodies and keeps us healthy

Root Cellar   An underground room that is a cooling system to keep roots (such as carrots and potatoes) from spoiling. Dug into the ground, this cellar acted as a refrigerator.

Saturated Fat   All animal fats – such as those in meat, poultry, and dairy – are saturated. Processed food and fast foods also are saturated. Also, tropical oils and palm kernel oil are highly saturated. Saturated fats are very unhealthy fat, clogging arteries and raising cholesterol, which can lead to heart disease

Stroke   A sudden, severe loss of muscle control and/or unconsciousness. This happens when a blood vessel in the brain is blocked or breaks.

Sucrose   Commonly called table sugar or granulated sugar; it is a refined sugar extracted from sugarcane and/or sugar beets

Supersize   A common expression in fast food restaurants meaning to make the portion of food/drink even larger

Supplement   Something added to improve one's diet, such as an herb or vitamin

Tendons   Cords of tough tissue that connect muscle to the bone

Tissue   A group of similar cells working together to perform a function, such
               As muscle tissue

Toxin   A poisonous, harmful, or unhealthy substance introduced into the
               body tissues – for example, grease from French fries. Toxins must be
               flushes from our bodies, by drinking water, or they can build up to a
               dangerous level

Toxin metals Poisonous metals such as mercury or copper that invade the body

Triglycerides Fats; produced by our bodies and stored as fat from excess calories
               from any source – protein, carbohydrates, or fats. Hormones
               regularly release triglycerides from fat tissue so provide energy, but
               an excess can cause coronary artery disease – a disease of the heart
               and arteries

Type 2 Diabetes The most common type of diabetes (also called adult-onset
               diabetes). This disease is caused when the body doesn't produce
               enough insulin or can't use the insulin it produces and blood sugar
               backs up in the blood stream.

Unsaturated Fats Also known as unsaturated triglyceride; unsaturated fats that
               come from corn, peanut, and olive oils; a good source fat and protein.

Vitamin   Substance that is found in food from plants and animals (for example,
               Dairy products, fruits and veggies) that keeps us healthy, builds strong
               bones, and helps us fight disease

Water-soluble Dissolved in water and quickly urinated

Index

Endorphins
Ephedra

F
Fast food
Fat
Fat cells
Fatigue
Fatty liver
Fawcett, Joy; also soccer
Fetal monitors
Fiber
Fibers
Fleming, Peggy
Flexibility
Flying, airlines
Food and Drug Administration (FDA)
Fructose

G
Glial cells
Gliding; hand gliding
Glucose
Golf

H
Handgliding or gliding
Handstands; also see yoga
Hanley, Linda; also volleyball
Harvard Medical School
Harvard University
Harvard University Nurses' Health Study
Headstands; also see yoga
Heart disease
Heart rate
Heart rate monitors
Heated pools
Heavy weight lifting; see weight lifting
Hepatitis
High altitude
High blood pressure

High impact exercise
Hike or hiking
Hip Hop; also see dance
Hormones
Horseback riding
Hot tubs
Hot yoga; also see yoga
House of Energy & Commerce Committee
Hunger pangs; also see eating or diet
Hydration
Hydroxycut
Hyperglycemia

I
Immune system
Insulin
Insulin surges or resistant
Intercourse; see lovemaking
Irregular periods; also see menstrual

J
Jogging; also see running
John Hopkins University
Joli, Angelina
Jones, Marion
Journal, how to write entries
Joyner, Florence Griffith
Jumping
Jumping rope

K
Kayaking
Kegel
Kickboxing
Kidneys
Kung fu; also martial arts

L
Labor & delivery
Lactid acid
Liquid candy or liquid drinks
Liver; also see fatty liver
Loma Linda University

Love making
Low impact exercise
Lunges; also squats

M

Macrominerals
Macronutrients
Martino, Angel; also see swimming
McCutchan, Lili
Memory, short-term
Memory; see muscle memory
Menstrual cycle
Mercury
Metabolism
Micromineral
Micronutrients
Minerals
Miscarriage
Models, role model
Models, supermodels
Monounsaturated fats
Moore, Demi
Mother fuel
Motorcycling
Morning sickness
Mountain biking
Muscle; building of
Muscle memory

N

National Academy of Science
Nordic ski
Nutritionist; also see dietician

O

Obesity
Ohio State University
Olenick, Mollee; also see pregnancy.org
Organic foods
Osteoporosis

Overweight
oxygen

P
Pilates
Pfeiffer, W.A.
Phosphates
Phytonutrients
Plyometrics
Pole vaulting
Polyunsaturated fats
Pool, also chlorine or hot tubs
Pores; also acne or skin
Post-partum depression
Power yoga; also see yoga
Pregnancy.org
Prenatal vitamins
Prenatal exercise
Prenatal yoga
Protein

R
Race; also see running
Race walking
Randolf Macon College
Reaching; also stretching
Rebound headaches
Rectal thermometer
Recovery of exercise
Recovery from childbirth
Reece, Gabrielle
Retton, Mary Lou
Reyes, Ernie
Rhee, Jhoon
Rock climbing
Rohl, Michelle; also race walking
Role model
Round ligaments
Royal Post Graduate Medical School
Running

Twisting; deep twisting

U
Underweight
University of California at Davis
University of London
University of Miami School of Medicine
University of Michigan
University of Richmond
Urine; frequency of and color of
Uterus
Uterus fundus

V
Vitamins
Vitamin C
Volleyball

W
Wakeboarding
Walking
Water; also see hydration
Water aerobics
Water retention; also bloat
Waterskiing
Water sports
Weather; also see air quality
Weight gain
Weight lifting
Weight loss
Whitewater rafting
World Health Organization

Y
Yale University
yoga

Welcome to the Mother Club!